the**facts**

Eating disorders

also available in thefacts series

the**facts**

Eating disorders

SIXTH EDITION

SUZANNE ABRAHAM

Associate Professor
Department of Women's Health
Royal North Shore Hospital
The University of Sydney
and
Co-Director of the Eating Disorders Unit
The Northside Clinic
The University of Sydney

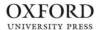

OXFORD
UNIVERSITY PRESS

OXFORD

UNIVERSITY PRESS

Great Clarendon Street, Oxford OX2 6DP

Oxford University Press is a department of the University of Oxford.
It furthers the University's objective of excellence in research, scholarship,
and education by publishing worldwide in

Oxford New York

Auckland Cape Town Dar es Salaam Hong Kong Karachi
Kuala Lumpur Madrid Melbourne Mexico City Nairobi
New Delhi Shanghai Taipei Toronto

With offices in

Argentina Austria Brazil Chile Czech Republic France Greece
Guatemala Hungary Italy Japan Poland Portugal Singapore
South Korea Switzerland Thailand Turkey Ukraine Vietnam

Oxford is a registered trade mark of Oxford University Press
in the UK and in certain other countries

Published in the United States
by Oxford University Press Inc., New York

© Oxford University Press 2008

The moral rights of the author have been asserted
Database right Oxford University Press (maker)

First published 1984
Sixth edition 2008

British Library Cataloguing in Publication Data
Data available

Library of Congress Cataloguing in Publication Data
Abraham, Suzanne.
  Eating disorders: the facts/Suzanne Abraham.—6th ed.
    p. cm.—(The facts)
  ISBN–13: 978–0–19–955101–9
1. Eating disorders. 2. Bulimia. I. Title.
  RC552.E18A27 2008
616.85'26—dc22

                                        2008019082

Typeset in Cepha Imaging Pvt. Ltd., Bangalore, India
Printed in China
through Asia Pacific Offset

ISBN 978-0-19-955101-9 (Pbk.)

1 3 5 7 9 10 8 6 4 2

Preface and acknowledgements

This book is written for patients, their families, and health professionals, particularly family doctors. More and more women are seeking help for their eating disorder, and most women who want treatment have a mixture of eating-disorder behaviours and characteristics that do not always fulfil the diagnostic criteria for anorexia nervosa or bulimia nervosa. They may have features of both or also be obese. This does not mean that they only have a mild disorder; they may be very physically unwell and have a poor quality of life.

At present, there is no easy way of classifying the eating disorders. It is probably easier to think of one eating disorder with different characteristics. I have chosen in this book to classify the eating disorders as (1) anorexia nervosa and anorexia nervosa-like disorders; (2) bulimia nervosa and bulimia nervosa-like disorders; and (3) obesity and overeating disorders. I hope this will allow readers to select the features that are relevant for them at the time from the different sections.

I wanted the new format of this 6th edition to remain faithful to my original aims, which were: first, to provide accurate information that will allow people who suffer from eating and weight problems to obtain information that improves their quality of life, and secondly, to provide a balanced approach that is useful for the general practitioner, as they will be consulted by people with transitory, easily resolved problems as well as the chronic cases frequently portrayed in books or found on the Internet. The following questions are typical of those asked by carers of patients with eating disorders:

- What causes the illness?

- What do you do to make her better?

- How can we help her?

- Should we comment on her eating and weight?

- Should you say anything when her behaviour is unacceptable?

- Why can't she eat?

- Why can't she stop eating?

- Will she ever get better or will she always have an eating disorder?

- How long will she need treatment?

- Will her bones recover?

- Will her heart and kidneys be permanently damaged?

- Has the family caused the eating disorder?

- Is it genetic?

- Will she be able to have children?

- Is it because her grandmother suffered depression?

- Will she ever be her old self again?

- Do you ever really recover from an eating disorder?

I have attempted to answer these questions as fully as possible in this book.

Nowadays most people with eating disorders recover and maintain a good quality of life. They frequently form relationships and desire children; and if they are not achieving pregnancy they will seek assisted conception. Not a lot is known about disordered eating and pregnancy. The chapter on pregnancy and the postpartum period addresses many issues including the challenge of pregnancy and the possible outcomes for both mothers and their babies.

In this 6th edition I would like to thank Christine Allwang and Angela Walker. They have provided their expertise as well as the more mundane work involved in the complete revision, rewrite and reformat of the book. **Eating Disorders: The Facts** could never have been written without discussions and help from our colleagues and friends. They include: Janice Russell, Susan Hart, Catherine Boyd, Jim Telfer, Michael Mira, Janet Conti, Sarah Maguire, Amanda McBride, David Blythe, Georgina Luscombe, Astrid von Lojewski, and the staff at the eating disorders unit at the Northside Clinic, Greenwich.

Most of all I would like to thank our patients. Without them there would be no book. I would particularly like to thank those patients who permitted us to use their emails, letters and diaries (appropriately modified for reason of privacy) for the case histories and quotations.

This book is not intended to glamorize or sensationalize eating disorders. I have presented the facts in the key points at the beginning of each chapter and highlighted others throughout the book. Some suggestions have also been added that will allow people to help themselves in conjunction with their usual treatment.

Note

Because of problems of gender in the English language, and because we treat more women than men with eating disorders we have chosen to use 'she' rather than 'he' in most cases.

The generally accepted measure of body thinness and fatness is body mass index (BMI kg/m^2) (Appendix A). Conversion for height and weight units is given in Appendices A and B.

Contents

1

Adolescent eating behaviour

➡ Key points

◆ Before menstruation, a woman's energy intake increases as unknown factors stimulate her to eat more

◆ There is a body weight challenge for women following first menstruation

◆ Women's concerns over their body weight, shape, and appearance increase after first menstruation and these are accompanied by a loss of self-esteem and increase in feelings of anxiety, depression, and social unease

◆ Between one-third and two-thirds of all teenage women in developed countries go on diets, with one in six adolescents dieting seriously

◆ Control around food is easier early in the menstrual cycle

'If I was going to get a job when I left school, I felt I had to be lighter. All my friends were dieting but my mother disapproved. She said it was puppy fat which would disappear. I knew it wouldn't, so I had to pretend I was not hungry because I wanted to be slim.'

History of body appearance

For most of recorded history, a woman was seen as desirable when her body was plump due to the deposition of fat on her breasts, hips, thighs, and abdomen. It was fashionable to be fat. The cultural belief that to be fat was to be attractive was due to the uncertainty of food supplies in pre-industrial and early industrial societies, to the irregular occurrence of famines, and to the effects of diseases, which eliminated large numbers of farm labourers. A curvaceous female body indicated that the husband (or father) was prudent,

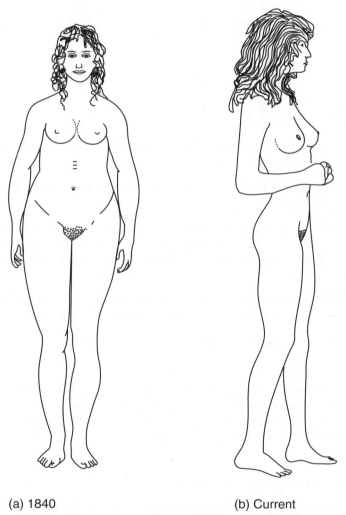

(a) 1840   (b) Current

Figure 1.1 The changing fashion in women's figures. The first illustration is taken from an obstetrical textbook printed in England in 1840, the second from a current textbook

efficient, and affluent. It also indicated that the woman was prepared for times of food shortage. Her family would be protected because she had sufficient energy, stored in her body in the form of fat, to look after her family.

Over the past 75 years, with abundant food supplies and good food distribution in most of the developed nations of the Western world, almost for the first time in history slimness has begun to be fashionable. This is documented in fashion magazines, in *Playboy* centrefolds, and in records of the 'vital statistics' of women winning beauty contests. For the past three decades, the public perception has been that a woman is attractive, desirable, and successful when she is slim. Fashion models have become taller and thinner, and have body weights at least 20% less than a woman of similar age and height living in a consumer society (Figure 1.1).

Over the same period of time, the body weight of men and women of all ages has risen and is continuing to increase at alarming rates in Westernized and less-developed countries. Obesity is considered the major global health problem of this century. Not surprisingly, this has led governments worldwide to consult their public health experts and produce guidelines for 'healthy eating and exercise as a way of life'.

A major global health message is to be or to become thin, and to look and be 'fit and healthy'. The messages 'to lose weight' and 'to be fit and healthy' particularly influence teenage women at a time in their life when they are undergoing emotional stress as they seek to achieve independence from their parents, to compete with their peers, and to find their identity. Adolescence is a time of concern about appearance. They believe that achieving the ideal body image will ensure success and happiness.

Growth spurts and body image changes during puberty

In late childhood, hormonal changes trigger an increase in height in girls and boys. This increase, or growth spurt, occurs at an earlier age in girls than in boys and is achieved by the child increasing the amount of food he or she eats (Figure 1.2). In girls, the onset of the growth spurt precedes the onset of menstruation.

There is a wide time range in the onset and duration of the growth spurt, and the peak may be reached by girls as early as 10 years of age or as late as 15. The growth spurt is accompanied by marked changes in the bodily appearance of the two sexes, which in turn are dependent on the sex hormones that

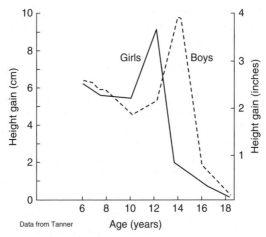

Figure 1.2 The spurt in growth at puberty

are now being produced in the girl's ovaries or the boy's testicles. Girls have a particularly large spurt in hip growth, resulting in widening of the hips.

Fat is also deposited beneath the skin, in the breasts, and over the hips. Obviously the amount of fat deposited is related to the energy absorbed from the food the girl eats and is influenced by the hormonal changes that are occurring at this time. During early adolescence, unknown factors stimulate the teenager to eat more, with the consequence that the energy intake for girls reaches a maximum during the age range of 11–14, at a time when her energy needs are great. From about the age of 14, a teenage girl's energy needs fall, but if she continues to eat the same amount as she has been eating, she will absorb an excess of energy, which will be converted into fat, and she may gain weight.

 Fact!

In contrast to boys, girls do not lose fat during the growth spurt.

Girls have a tendency to increase their body fat, particularly on the upper legs, as they cease to gain height.

At puberty, both sexes show an increase in muscle bulk, but this is much more marked in boys.

Body weight after the first menstrual period (menarche)

A clearer picture of the weight challenge young women experience emerges if we look at when women have their first menstrual period rather than their age. Recently, we measured the height and weight of over 300 girls aged 11–16 and asked them about the weight they would like to be, how they felt about their body appearance, and how many months it had been since their first menstruation.

 Fact!

Women gain weight following first menstruation.

Women have a poorer body image after first menstruation.

Body mass index (BMI) was calculated from the student's height and weight measurements (see page 22) and is shown in Figure 1.3. In the 6–12 months

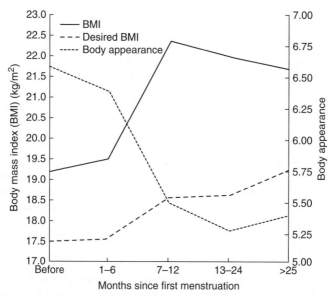

Figure 1.3 BMI, desired BMI, and increasing negative feelings about body appearance (on a scale of 0–10) following first menstruation

after a woman has her first period, there is an increase in BMI, almost all of which is due to a rapid rise in body weight, although women are still growing a small amount in height at this time. The decreasing BMI that occurred more than a year after first menstruation suggests that these students had changed their eating and exercise habits and lifestyles, some because they were responding to their bodies altered energy needs while others were starting to use methods of weight loss at this time.

The students desired BMI, which is the weight they would like to be for their height, and their rating of their body appearance (out of 10, with 10 being the best) are shown in Figure 1.3. At all times, they wanted their body weight to be less than their actual weight and did not like their body appearance as much after their weight gain in the year after first menstruation.

This is the adolescent girl's dilemma. She may wish to remain thin or to become thin, because cultural norms expect her to be thin, or she may reject those norms, either because of conflict within herself or within her family, or because she enjoys and finds emotional release in eating. If she chooses to become and remain thin, she has to learn new eating habits that provide a balance between her energy input and her energy needs (output). This can be a challenge for the adolescent woman.

Changes in self-esteem during adolescence

In the early stages of puberty and before first menstruation, most girls feel good about themselves. They feel content with their relationships, their family and friends, their school life, their performance, and how they look. In other words, they have a high self-esteem. As a girl's growth spurt comes to an end and her first menstrual period occurs, her self-esteem and feelings about her body appearance decline (Figure 1.3).

It is these changes around first menstruation, including weight gain, that are accompanied by a loss of confidence and a decrease in self-esteem among young women. Not only is their opinion of their body appearance poorer, but their overall self-esteem is lower; this includes the areas of self-esteem that are valued most by young women, which are relating well to others and having close relationships, doing well at school or work, and being romantically attractive to others.

Young men are different. In a recent study of pre- and post-pubertal male and female school students, we found that post-pubertal male students had the greatest self-esteem and female post-pubertal students the lowest. There was a big discrepancy between what young women feel they 'should be like' and how they 'feel they are'. In other words, young women in their early teens already feel they have failed to reach their expectations of themselves, whereas young men are fulfilling their expectations of themselves.

 Fact!

Young women experience a decrease in their self-esteem after first menstruation.

Young men experience an increase in their self-esteem as they grow taller, become heavier, and increase their muscle mass.

Being overweight and obese in the teenage years also affects students' self-esteem. Overweight young people, both male and female students, have a lower self-esteem than their normal-weight male and female peers.

Anxiety, depression, and adolescence

Accompanying the changes in self-esteem are changes in other psychological characteristics. A large epidemiological study found that there was an increase in feelings of depression and anxiety during adolescence for both young men and young women. This change was greatest for young women at the time of first menstruation. The results led the researchers to conclude that '*menarche marks a transition in the risk for depression and anxiety in young women*'.

One particular type of anxiety called 'social anxiety' becomes apparent during puberty. The main feature of social anxiety is a fear of embarrassment or humiliation in social situations where the person worries that others are judging their performance. It is a fear of failing in front of others. This can occur when people are eating or speaking in front of other people and in the classroom when someone watches them working. The sufferer may avoid eye contact with people, blush, stop what they are doing, and appear generally anxious.

 Fact!

Feeling anxious around people, particularly people you do not know well, is a common worry of people with eating problems.

Attitudes to diet after first menstruation

Until a few months before a woman's first period, she usually does not think about dieting and if she is asked the question 'What does dieting mean?', she is likely to describe dieting as 'healthy eating'. It is not until she has grown taller, menstruated, and increased her body weight that her perception of dieting includes the idea that dieting is for loss of body weight (see box below). Prepubertal girls who report dieting for weight loss have usually been advised to lose weight and exercise by their school as they have been classified as over-weight or obese, while others are shown how to diet by their older sister or mother as they wish to avoid becoming like family members who are overweight or obese. Frequently, they 'diet with' their sister or mother and understand dieting to be a lifestyle that is continued throughout life.

Responses of 13-year-old students trying to lose body weight when asked, 'Is dieting different after your first period?'

- 'Dieting becomes more serious and you think about it more.'

- 'You start to get more interested [in yourself].'

- 'I put on stacks of weight.'

- 'You feel you're getting fat. I don't want to turn out like my stepmum.'

- 'After your period you worry about your appearance.'

- 'I worry what people think—mostly boys.'

- 'Don't know, I've only had one period.'

- 'I try to lose weight for my boyfriend.'

- 'My sister's friend was anorexic. She didn't get periods. She stopped eating to stop her periods.'

Over-perception of body size

A young woman's perception of her body is important to her psychological well-being. She may see her body as overweight, unhealthy, and unfit compared with those of fashionable and popular media personalities. The over-perception of body size is found among teenage girls in many countries. Nine studies on the perception of body size of teenage women from Sweden, the USA, and Australia have been conducted over the decades ranging from the 1960s to the present. The investigations showed that between one-third and one-half of teenagers whose weight was normal perceived themselves to be overweight, and three-quarters wanted to lose weight. These percentages have remained constant over each decade.

Like Swedish and American teenagers, most Australian women want to lose more weight from certain parts of their body. When asked, from where do you want to lose weight, their answers were:

- Thighs 64%

- Bottom 45%

- Hips 43%

- Waist/stomach 22%

- Legs 20%

- Face 9%

- All over 9%

- Breasts 6%

- Arms 6%.

Body image after first menstruation

Young women's concerns about their body weight, body shape, and body appearance increase in the year after their first period. In response to these worries, most women commence dieting, exercising, or trying to reduce their food intake. A few years later, these young teenagers appear to adjust and become more accepting of their increased body weight but not their body appearance. Their body image concerns continue to increase along with psychological changes in anxiety, depression, social unease, and feelings of loss of control following first menstruation. The development of all of these worries, feelings, and dieting behaviour from the time of first menstruation are shown in Figure 1.4.

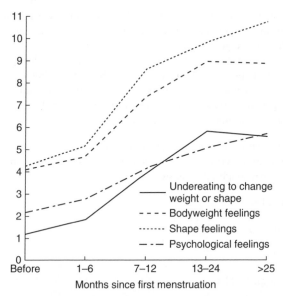

Figure 1.4 Increasing negative feelings (on a scale of 0–20) about body shape and weight and dieting following first menstruation

Eating and the menstrual cycle

In two studies, we found evidence to support an association between the menstrual cycle and food intake in young women.

◆ There is an increase in intake of carbohydrates, protein, fats, and hence of energy in the few days before and after the onset of bleeding.

◆ Individual women show a wide variation in the amount of food eaten, frequently depending on how the woman is feeling.

◆ Many women have feelings of depression, irritability, and tension just before their period.

◆ Women enjoy a feeling of well-being and a decrease in their appetite in the week after menstruation.

Women find dieting and control around food more difficult between ovulation and menstruation (premenstrum).

Fact!

It is easier to diet and control your eating in the week after your period.

Usually, the greater the food restriction early in the menstrual cycle, the more likely that a craving for food will result in overeating or binge eating in the premenstrual phase of that menstrual cycle.

Adolescent eating and weight-losing behaviour

Faced with the belief that they are overweight, it appears that between one-third and two-thirds of all teenage women in the USA and similar developed countries go on diets and that one woman in six diets 'seriously'.

Table 1.1 Behaviours present among secondary and tertiary students and patients with eating disorders in the previous month (aged 13–25)

Behaviours present in last 28 days	Students (n=440)	Patients with eating disorders (n=130)
Trying to lose weight	66	84
Restricting food intake	49	83
Restricting food intake >14 days	29	84
Exercise for shape/weight	56	62
Excessive exercise for any reason[a]	15	24
Excessive exercise >19 days[a]	7	14
Binge eating[b]	16	44
Binge eating >1/week	6	24
Chewing and spitting out food	1	11
Self-induced vomiting	7	37
Laxative misuse	2	18
Purging (vomiting/laxatives) >1/week	4	42
Smoking cigarettes for weight	10	20
Drinking coffee for weight	4	23
Slimming tablets	4	8
Social drugs for weight	3	7

[a] >500 kcal.

[b] Binge eating: episodes of eating large amounts of food and feeling out of control.

In four Australian studies of young women aged 13–25, from 1980 to the present, the findings have been very similar. Most women had tried to diet at some time, the majority first trying between the ages of 13 and 18. Most said that they wanted to be a little or a lot lighter in weight and one-third said they had difficulty in controlling their weight. Their behaviour over the past month is given in Table 1.1. The only difference in the numbers of women employing these behaviours in the twenty-first century compared with the twentieth century is the introduction of social 'party' drugs (Table 1.1). The weight control measures described by these healthy women are also used by women who have an eating disorder.

Table 1.2 Weight-losing behaviour of 300 healthy women

Weight-losing behaviour	Aged 10–14 (%)	Aged 15–25 (%)
Avoiding eating between meals	73	78
Exercising (usually alone)	44	75
Dieting—'own diet'	35	55
Avoiding eating breakfast	–	48
Keeping busy to avoid temptation to eat	38	46
Selecting low-energy foods	32	41
Counting calories/kilojoules	–	34
Avoiding situations where food is offered	15	25
Dieting with a friend	–	22
Using illness as an excuse not to eat	–	21
Exercising with a friend	–	20
Drinking water before eating	29	18
Taking 'natural' laxatives	11	16
Lying about amount of food eaten	–	16
Weighing self several times a day	4	15
Smoking cigarettes	2	14
Dieting—magazine diet	16	12
Keeping no food at home	–	12
Avoiding eating with family	1	10

Many young women start trying simple and safe methods of weight control, such as not snacking between meals and exercising (Table 1.2). By the age of 15 or 16, young women may commence dieting for shorter or longer periods, with about a quarter of those who diet doing so 'seriously'.

By the age of 18, on average, a minority of adolescent women who are having serious problems with eating, body shape, and body weight may try more extreme methods of weight control, such as fasting for a day or two, to try to reduce their weight quickly, or trying self-induced vomiting and laxative abuse. These more serious behaviours usually first occur by the age of 22. As well as restricting food intake and exercising to lose weight, a number of women go on eating binges, usually starting at around the age of 18.

Media, the Internet, and school influences

Magazines, the media, the Internet, and schools all provide information that may contribute to the development of an eating disorder. Also implicated are the advertising, fitness, and food industries. The media and fashion industry have been 'blamed' for causing eating disorders by promoting the sylph-like figures of models as the ideal body image. For a few women this can be a trigger, but most young teenagers are now much more discerning about what they see and read in the media; for example, they know the tricks used by photographers of teen models in the production of fashion magazines. They know that most women can never become a model, even with the help of an 'extreme makeover'.

All sources of information can appear to trigger the development of an eating disorder in a teenager. For example, when an already slim teenager learns that 'it is healthy to eat less fat and do more exercise', they may begin to lose weight and develop anorexia nervosa, while the message that 'you are from a genetically obese family' may allow an already overweight teenager to ignore good eating messages and accept obesity.

The message that 'exercise is healthy and more exercise is healthier' is being promoted by health experts and the fitness industry. Currently, there is no information about how exercise may be unhealthy and when the amount is considered to be excessive, except on the Internet. When energy intake in the form of food is not sufficient to meet the needs of the body and the energy expended during exercise, this can not only result in the loss of menstrual periods, but may also, if sustained, trigger the onset of an eating disorder or compulsive exercise disorder (see Chapter 2).

Smoking and body weight

At a time when the health risks of smoking are becoming increasingly apparent, the use of cigarette smoking by young women as a method of weight control is not decreasing. Although the number of Australian female teenagers who are classified as 'current smokers' has decreased from 20 to 15%; unfortunately the number who use smoking to control their weight remains around 12%. Findings in the UK and USA suggest that the greater the concern a young woman has about her weight, the greater is her use of cigarettes. In a study of pregnant women we conducted on two occasions 20 years apart, we found that 4% of the women continued to smoke during pregnancy in order to control their weight gain, despite having been advised not to.

It is now thought that the weight gain after quitting smoking is a result of returning a person to their normal body weight. Tobacco smoking is thought to cause an artificially lower body weight for a variety of physiological and psychological reasons. Possible reasons for weight gain after stopping smoking are:

- Smoking may be a psychological substitute for eating.

- Nicotine may improve depressed moods (effect on chemicals in the brain, e.g. serotonin).

- Nicotine may suppress appetite (effect on chemicals in the brain, e.g. serotonin).

- Nicotine increases the basal metabolic rate (BMR), probably by increasing the amount of fat, protein, and glycogen used by the body and decreasing the amount of glucose taken into tissues of the body (nicotine reduces the release of the hormone insulin after food is eaten). An increase in BMR without an increase in food intake will result in weight decrease.

- Nicotine has a stimulatory effect and contributes to the overall lower body weight of smokers.

Promising recent studies from Germany suggest that, if women are aware that weight gain can follow smoking cessation, they can prevent it happening.

Binge eating and eating disorders

Some young women intersperse periods of strict dieting by episodes of uncontrollable overeating, or binge eating. The lack of energy available for normal body function sends messages to a centre in the brain, which increases the urge to eat, and often to overeat or binge. In most cases, the eating binges are infrequent and do not affect the young woman's quality of life or her lifestyle. In some cases, her psychological and physical health is affected as she battles to have control over her eating behaviour, which may result in the development of bulimia nervosa, particularly if she employs extreme methods of weight control. If she overeats with increasing frequency so that her energy intake exceeds her energy output she will become obese, and if she binge eats she may develop binge-eating disorder.

Other young women are so concerned about losing control of their eating behaviour and not being 'healthy' that they slowly restrict the foods they eat and start on a relentless pursuit of thinness. They eat minimal amounts of food and may exercise excessively, and some use extreme methods of weight control. The result is that they become emaciated and develop anorexia nervosa.

Although these disorders predominantly affect young women in Western countries, research shows that the same problems are being increasingly diagnosed among all ethnic groups, e.g. in Japan, Malaysia, China, and India.

The outcome of the young woman's concern about her body shape and her disordered eating behaviour is shown in Figure 1.5. The disordered eating behaviour usually starts between the ages of 14 and 18.

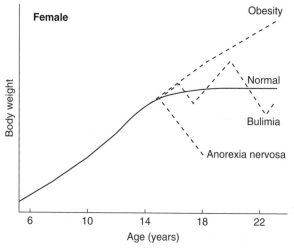

Figure 1.5 The onset of eating disorders

We would stress that anorexia nervosa, bulimia nervosa, binge-eating disorder and obesity are not *illnesses* in themselves. They become illnesses when they:

◆ interfere with the person's physical or mental comfort;

◆ are likely to produce medical complications;

◆ disorganize the person's life to a marked degree; or

◆ distort the person's life so that close relatives are also involved and help is sought.

In other words, they become disorders when the person's quality of life is affected. Unfortunately, in severe cases, unless treatment is sought, the eating disorder may lead to the premature death of the victim.

Table 1.3 Attitudes of 100 healthy pregnant women admitted consecutively to a teaching hospital to give birth to their first child (reported 3–5 days postpartum)

Behaviour	Attitude during pregnancy (%)
Eating and weight	
'Watched their weight'	71
Thoughts of food interfered with concentration	52
Preoccupied with thoughts of food	8
Binge eating	44
Binge eating a problem	9[a]
Problems controlling weight	41
Dangerous weight-losing behaviours	
Any one dangerous method	11
Excessive exercise	4
Smoking cigarettes (for weight loss)	4
Episodic starvation	3
Misuse of laxatives	2
Inducing vomiting (for weight loss)	1

[a] Three times more than before pregnancy.

Pregnancy and eating behaviour

Although most eating-disorder problems start in adolescence, a further challenge to some women's weight, body image, exercise routine, and eating behaviour may occur when they become pregnant (Table 1.3).

Because of their concern about weight gain, many of the women (Table 1.3) used one or more ways of controlling their weight gain. Most of the methods adopted were sensible, e.g. nearly half of the pregnant women reduced their food intake modestly by choosing low-energy foods, by avoiding eating between meals, or by exercising sensibly. Most of these women had used similar methods to control their weight before becoming pregnant.

Most women meet this challenge to their body image and adjust to the changes of pregnancy, childbirth, breastfeeding, and parenthood. Women who have 'normal eating patterns' frequently feel that they improve their eating patterns and nutrition during pregnancy, as they wish to care for their developing child. Being aware of the gain in body weight and the possibility of not losing this weight after the birth is a common concern of pregnancy. The experiences of pregnant women suffering from eating disorders are discussed in Chapter 4.

2

Eating disorders—an overview

⮕ Key points

- Women with eating disorders are preoccupied with thoughts of control over food, eating, or weight

- Anorexia nervosa disorders are characterized by weight loss and low body weight

- Bulimia nervosa disorders are characterized by binge eating and the use of extreme behaviour to prevent weight gain

- Eating disorders can be described as: high weight, low weight, vomiting, purging, binge eating, atypical exercise

- Onset of binge eating episodes are associated with anxiety, stress, and negative emotions

- Exercise rather than weight can be the focus of an eating disorder

'The human being is an open social system, each one, in its own way unique. My food problem is my somewhat unique reaction to a board of external and internal influences. Human beings prefer things in a state of organization, they dislike randomness and attempt to classify.'

Control of eating

The control of normal eating behaviour is not well understood. Although more is known about the many factors that influence the control of food intake, it is still puzzling how they all fit together. The discovery of leptin is an important recent advancement, as this hormone is involved in the energy balance in the body of humans. It is secreted by fat (adipose) tissue and reflects the amount of energy stored in the body as fat. The higher your body weight (fat), the higher the levels of leptin in your bloodstream.

 Fact!

Leptin tells the body when you are satiated (full) and do not need further food.

Ghrenlin tells the body when you need to eat.

Receptors in the hypothalamus of the brain are sensitive to the levels of leptin and regulate the amount of body fat by controlling the appetite and increasing energy output. The most potent appetite stimulant in the brain is called neuropeptide Y (NPY); leptin decreases appetite by suppressing NPY. Another hormone in the body called ghrenlin has the opposite effect and stimulates NPY. Other hormones released from the stomach, intestines, and bloodstream including insulin and cholecystokinin in turn regulate leptin and ghrenlin. Insulin is a messenger of satiation and is produced by the pancreas in response to an increase in blood glucose. Cholecystokinin is produced by the duodenum and is thought to regulate the size of the meal eaten.

How the sight, smell, and taste sensations associated with food are integrated with the chemical and neural messages received by the brain is unclear, as these sensations may encourage or discourage eating.

Women with eating disorders often believe 'you are what you eat' and believe that they can control their body weight by the food they eat. In fact, 75% of the energy derived from foodstuffs is converted into heat, which is used to keep the cells of the body warm so that each cell can carry out the work it is designed to do to help the body function as a whole. Which receptors in the brain keep body weight so surprisingly stable in most individuals is unknown. We do know that increased levels of leptin in the blood increase the body's activity and heat production (in addition to decreasing food intake), resulting in increased energy loss. This may account, at least in part, for the relative stability of body weight for most people. What is also known is that these mechanisms and receptors fail to function when they are over- or understimulated by starvation or by gorging and binge eating. Somehow these messages to and from the brain are scrambled by these behaviours. A genetic failure of release of the leptin is also implicated in some cases of obesity.

Fact!

Women with eating disorders feel that their perceptions of hunger and satiation (fullness) are not to be believed.

Defining an ideal weight

A number of calculations have been used to define maximum and minimum ideal weights. The simplest is a measurement of weight against height, as used by insurance companies (Figure 2.1). A more sophisticated measure takes into account the person's age, as well as weight and height, as obtained from a table prepared by the Society of Actuaries, and is called the average body weight (ABW).

The body mass index (BMI) is the third type of calculation and the one used in this book. Devised in 1871 by a Belgian astronomer and mathematician, Dr Quetelet, for defining obesity, it is equally valuable in reaching a diagnosis

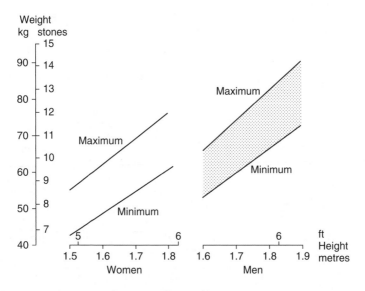

Figure 2.1 Maximum and minimum ideal weights for men and women of different heights wearing light clothing

of anorexia nervosa. The Quetelet Index, which is now known as the BMI, is calculated from the simple formula:

$$\frac{\text{weight (kg)}}{\text{height (m)} \times \text{height (m)}} \text{ kg/m}^2$$

The person is weighed in indoor clothing without shoes (Figure 2.2). A table of heights and corresponding BMI values is available in Appendix A.

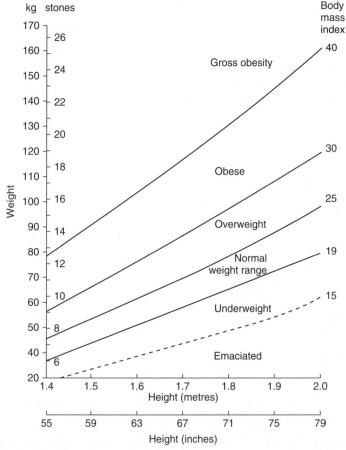

Figure 2.2 Body mass index (BMI kg/m²)

Anorexia nervosa

'People may find it hard to believe or comprehend why a person, supposedly intelligent and quite attractive and with a good family upbringing, would throw it all away for an obsessive need—no, desire!—to be slender and praised for the will-power to diet so well and easily.'

The term anorexia nervosa was first used by an English physician, Sir William Gull, in 1873. He described a young woman, 'Miss A', whom he had first seen 7 years earlier:

Her emaciation was very great. It was stated that she had lost 33 lbs. in weight. She was then 5 st. 12 lbs. Height, 5 ft. 5 in. Amenorrhoea for nearly a year. No cough. Respirations throughout chest everywhere normal. Heart sounds normal. Resp. 12; pulse, 56. No vomiting nor diarrhoea. Slight constipation. Complete anorexia for animal food, and almost complete anorexia for everything else. Abdomen shrunk and flat, collapsed. No abnormal pulsations of aorta. Tongue clean. Urine normal. Slight deposit of phosphates on boiling. The condition was one of simple starvation. There was but slight variation in her condition, though observed at intervals of three or four months . . . The case was regarded as one of simple anorexia.

Various remedies were prescribed but no perceptible effect followed their administration. The diet also was varied, but without any effect upon the appetite. Occasionally for a day or two the appetite was voracious, but this was very rare and exceptional. The patient complained of no pain, but was restless and active. This was in fact a striking expression of the nervous state, for it seemed hardly possible that a body so wasted could undergo the exercise which seemed agreeable. There was some peevishness of temper, and a feeling of jealousy. No account could be given of the exciting cause. Miss A remained under my observation from January 1866 to March 1868, when she had much improved, and gained weight from 82 to 128 lbs. The improvement from this time continued, and I saw no more of her medically . . .

Sir William was in error: patients with anorexia nervosa do not have a lack of appetite. They are often hungry, but suppress their hunger and refuse to eat normally because of their relentless desire to be thin, even to the point of becoming emaciated, and their fear that they will lose control of their eating behaviour.

Main features of anorexia nervosa

The diagnostic criteria for anorexia nervosa are outlined in the box below.

Current diagnostic criteria for anorexia nervosa

◆ An intense fear of gaining weight or becoming fat, even though the woman is underweight

◆ Refusal to maintain her body weight in the normal weight range for her age and height; this is not due to any physical or mental disorder

◆ A BMI equal to or less than 17.5

◆ A disturbance in the perception of her body weight, size, or shape

◆ Denial about the serious nature of her current low body weight

◆ If she has entered her reproductive years (i.e. has passed puberty), no menstrual periods (amenorrhoea) for at least 3 consecutive months

Two types of anorexia nervosa have been suggested: restricting type and binge eating/purging type.

Modified from the *American Psychiatric Association: Diagnostic and Statistical and Manual of Mental Disorders*, 4th edn (2000), American Psychiatric Association, Washington DC. By permission.

Weight loss

When presenting to a doctor, the woman has usually lost a considerable amount of weight, so that her BMI is 17.5 kg/m^2 or below. Once a physical or a mental illness has been excluded as a possible cause for the low body weight, a woman whose BMI is less than 17.5 is likely to have anorexia nervosa.

The BMI of prepubertal girls must be interpreted carefully as no accurate BMI tables that include age are available. Teenage girls who have not started menstruating have lower BMIs than girls of the same age who have menstruated (Figure 2.3). Using 85% of expected body weight for age and height is generally appropriate for children.

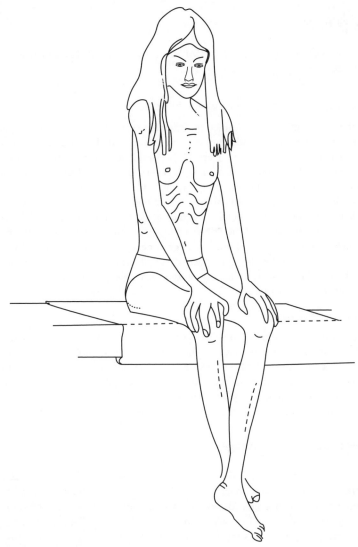

Figure 2.3 A young woman suffering from anorexia nervosa

Fact!

Asian women usually have a BMI value about one BMI point below Caucasian women.

Preoccupation with thoughts of weight or food

In the pursuit of thinness, women must remain ever vigilant in their quest and they become obsessed with thinking and planning their eating and weight-losing behaviour. The more starved the brain, the more obsessional the thoughts and behaviour become. They fear loss of control of their weight and their eating except at very low body weights, at BMIs of less than 15.5 kg/m², if at all. Thoughts about control over their body, food intake, activity, and weight-losing behaviours dictate how they live every moment of their life and it becomes increasingly difficult for them to separate their eating-disordered thoughts from their own thoughts. They appear to become consumed with their eating disorder to the point where they will cheat and lie to maintain their behaviour. *Preoccupation with eating-disordered thoughts interferes with their concentration on other things.*

Lack of menstruation

The third main feature of anorexia nervosa is that a girl who has started to menstruate ceases menstruating—she develops amenorrhoea. Most women cease to menstruate when their weight is in the BMI range of 17–19 kg/m² when they no longer have sufficient reserves of energy in their body to support a healthy pregnancy. If a woman is taking the oral contraceptive 'pill' or 'hormone replacement', this feature cannot be determined (see Chapter 7).

Perception of body image

'Before I started to lose weight, common sense tells me that my weight was not heavy for that height. But common sense had left me and I wanted to weigh about 43 kg (95 lb or 6 st 11 lb). And I achieved it! The strange thing is that whenever I went to buy new clothes, I always saw how revoltingly thin my image in the mirror actually was. But I still felt fat.'

Some experts claim that a distorted body image—the woman perceiving her body as larger, wider, and fatter than it is in reality—is a specific feature of anorexia nervosa. This is inaccurate, as many other women, such as pregnant women, who have recently changed their body shape have the same disturbed

Table 2.1 What young women would like their weight to be

Preferred weight	Healthy women (%) (n=106)	Ballet dancers (%) (n=50)	Anorexia nervosa patients (%) (n=22)	Bulimia nervosa patients (%) (n=44)
A lot heavier	0	1	9	0
A little heavier	1	1	50	0
Present weight	19	5	5	15
A little lighter	48	62	23	20
A lot lighter	32	31	13	65

body image. Many women who have normal eating behaviour also overestimate their body size, and in some cases overestimate it considerably more than women who have anorexia nervosa, especially when looking at their hip width and their body from the side. We found this over-perception of size among various different women when we asked the question 'What would you prefer your weight to be?' The groups were women who were students, ballet dancers, or had eating disorders. Each of the groups wanted to be thinner, except for over half of the patients with anorexia nervosa who were already at a very low weight (Table 2.1).

It is also possible that some of the reports that say that a distorted body image is a specific feature of anorexia nervosa may be due to the patient deceiving the doctor, as in the *Patient's perspective* below.

 Patient's perspective

'I've spoken to other anorexics and they realize just as I realize that at our lowest weights, we all knew we were damn thin. You'd have to be pretty stupid to think that you were not, but you have to hide it because if you let on to the doctors that you know you are thin, they will want to put weight on you. I won't tell my doctor though, because I want to stay like this: I feel safe, out of the world and men are too scared to touch me in case they break me. So I tell him, "Of course I'm not thin."'

Like other teenagers, women who have anorexia nervosa look at parts of their body, rather than at their body as a whole, when they look at themselves in a mirror (page 9). They see their abdomen as 'bulgy' and they want it to be flat, and their thighs as large and heavy, and may want them to be smooth and thinner.

It is true that many severely emaciated women suffering from anorexia nervosa lose insight into how emaciated they are and describe themselves as 'feeling fat'. 'Feeling fat' is frequently associated with feeling bad, with being worthless and unhappy. *Anorexia nervosa patients can differentiate between 'feeling fat' and 'looking fat'.*

Bulimia nervosa

'Looking back on the reason I started binge eating, I think it was because of my obsession with dieting. And that stemmed from the fact that I thought I was overweight when in reality I was short and had inherited fatter arms and legs than the average person.'

Bulimia means 'to eat like an ox'. Although people have been known to 'eat like oxen' from antiquity, it was not until 1979 that a London psychiatrist, Gerald Russell, identified 40% of his patients with anorexia nervosa with an 'ominous variation' of the disorder, the variation being that they periodically went on eating binges.

By 1982, it became clear that women who had never been at a low body weight also binge ate. As well as feeling that they have a lack of control over their eating behaviour, sufferers binge eat very frequently and adopt measures, some of which are extreme, to prevent themselves becoming increasingly fat.

Bulimic women were found to divide their days into 'good days' when they had no compulsion to binge eat and 'bad days' when they found the need to binge eat irresistible. They were also aware that anxiety, boredom, stress, or unhappiness could precipitate an episode of binge eating. *Bulimic women associate unpleasant feelings with the onset of a binge-eating episode.*

Features of bulimia nervosa

The diagnostic features of bulimia nervosa are outlined in the box below.

Current diagnostic criteria for bulimia nervosa

The woman:

- has recurrent episodes of binge eating, i.e. she rapidly consumes a large amount of food in a short period of time (usually less than 2 hours);

- feels that she lacks control over her eating behaviour during the eating binges;

- regularly engages in measures to prevent gaining weight, such as self-induced vomiting, misuse of laxatives or diuretics, strict dieting, fasting, or vigorous exercise;

- has had a minimum average of two binge-eating episodes a week (and the weight-gain prevention measures) for at least 3 months;

- has a persistent over-concern with her body shape and weight; and

- the eating disturbance does not occur exclusively in association with anorexia nervosa.

Two subtypes of bulimia nervosa have been suggested: purging and non-purging subtypes.

Modified from the *American Psychiatric Association: Diagnostic and Statistical Manual of Mental Disorders*, 4th edn (2000), American Psychiatric Association, Washington DC. By permission.

 Fact!

The features of patients with anorexia nervosa and bulimia nervosa are similar.

Fear of weight gain

Between binges, bulimia nervosa sufferers try to diet rigorously and may try to resist the urge to binge eat, rather as an alcoholic tries to resist the urge to drink (at least 20% of patients with bulimia nervosa also abuse alcohol or drugs). Most resort to more extreme methods such as inducing themselves to vomit, taking large amounts of laxatives in the belief that the food eaten will not be absorbed, or using stimulant and 'party' drugs. A minority of binge eaters do not induce vomiting and maintain a very strict diet between eating binges, controlling their weight in this way. They may find that eating 'anything' leads to binge eating and they alternate starvation with binge eating. *A woman with bulimia nervosa is aware that binge eating and overeating are different.*

Preoccupation with thoughts of food and control of body weight

Eating is a temporary way of escaping from these thoughts and the unpleasant stresses of life. The feelings of unhappiness, anxiety, or stress that precipitated an eating binge are relieved to a greater extent among those patients with bulimia nervosa who induce vomiting than among those who use other behaviours to avoid weight gain.

Binge eating

Binge eating occurs when the woman's resistance to eating fails and she has an irresistible desire to eat. This leads her to ingest excessive amounts of food, far more than is needed to maintain good nutrition and far more than most other people in her culture normally eat. This causes her to be secretive about her binge eating, at least in the early stages of the illness. Attempts by others to prevent her binge eating may be met by hostility.

Atypical or eating disorders not otherwise specified

Features of 'eating disorder not otherwise specified'

◆ If female: all of the criteria for anorexia nervosa are met, except that the woman menstruates regularly

◆ All of the criteria for anorexia nervosa are met except that, despite significant weight loss, the person's current weight is in the normal range

◆ All of the criteria for bulimia nervosa are met except that the binge eating and inappropriate behaviours (i.e. purging, laxative abuse, etc.) occur less than twice a week or for a duration of less than 3 months

♦ The person's weight is in the normal range, but they regularly induce vomiting after eating small amounts of food

♦ The person repeatedly chews and spits out large amounts of food rather than swallowing the food

Modified from the *American Psychiatric Association: Diagnostic and Statistical Manual of Mental Disorders*, 4th edn (2000), American Psychiatric Association, Washington DC. By permission.

Physicians who specialize in evaluating and treating patients with eating disorders find that many of their patients do not fulfil all of the criteria for a diagnosis of either bulimia nervosa or anorexia nervosa, and they are not obese. This does not mean that their eating disorder is less severe. They are given a diagnosis of 'eating disorder not otherwise specified' (EDNOS) following the advice of the American Psychiatric Association. Those women who can best be described as 'chaotic eaters', with a seemingly unpredictable collection of eating and weight-losing behaviours, are included in this classification.

Some of the women falling into this category may be in the process of:

♦ developing all of the features needed for a diagnosis of bulimia nervosa or anorexia nervosa;

♦ recovering from bulimia nervosa or anorexia nervosa;

♦ relapsing;

♦ proceeding from one eating disorder diagnosis to a different eating disorder diagnosis; or

♦ becoming obsessed with exercise rather than body weight.

Exercise disorder

This covers women with eating disorders who describe themselves as exercising to control their weight, to control their mood, and to be fit and healthy (Table 2.2).

I have used the term 'exercise disorder' to refer to behaviour and thinking about exercise that is unhealthy and has a negative impact on someone's quality of life. The term was first used in 1990 to refer to women who were

Table 2.2 Reasons for exercising given by people with exercise disorder

Reasons for exercise		
Mood	**Weight**	**Health**
To relieve anxious feelings	To lose weight	To be physically healthy
To relieve depressed feelings	To stop feeling guilty	To feel active
To stop feeling agitated	To burn energy	To stay in exercise routine
To block out unpleasant feelings	To feel thin	To help concentration
To relieve stress	To prevent weight gain	For a sense of achievement
To relieve anger/aggression	To feel in control	To feel good

seeking assisted conception because they were unable to modify their exercise to achieve pregnancy.

People with an exercise disorder usually:

◆ feel they must exercise (compulsively);

◆ feel preoccupied with thoughts of exercise that affect their concentration on other things;

◆ feel irritated or angry if their exercise is interrupted;

◆ do excessive amounts of exercise (for their health and injury status);

◆ allow exercise to take precedence over relationships and over most other daily activities;

◆ usually have to increase the amount of exercise to obtain the same effect; and

◆ are unable to stop exercising without physical and psychological 'withdrawal symptoms' of restlessness, agitation, or anger.

Approximately 15% of women with a normal-weight eating disorder also have an exercise disorder. The duration of an exercise disorder can be a few months to years. Currently, it is not known how many women have an exercise disorder after they have recovered from their eating disorder, or how many people in the community have an exercise disorder and have never had an eating disorder. A 'guestimate' would be less than 1%.

Patient's perspective

Belinda suffered from bulimia nervosa. For the past 3 years, she has maintained a BMI of 22 and is happy with her appearance. Her eating patterns are normal and she no longer binge eats, but she is a compulsive exerciser.

'Each day of my life, I try to fit my day around at least one session of quite strenuous, routine exercising—usually either 20 laps of a 50 metre pool or a 45 minute strenuous aerobic workout.

If I cannot fit in my usual daily piece of exercise, I feel guilty, worried, and up to a point anxious. Exercise has become an important part of my life. I should say that the main reason I exercise is for the actual feeling of being fit and feeling relaxed, not because I want to lose weight or look thin. I like me as I am now.

I do have the will-power to reduce exercising to only one session a day, but I push myself to it, even if my body just wants to flop. Afterwards, I feel really happy, even though I didn't enjoy doing it at the time. I feel so sick of it all, but would feel so unhappy and insecure if I stopped altogether. When I am emotionally upset over something important to me, I punish my body even more severely and increase the exercise. I feel weakness and no strength during an exercise session but I cannot stop doing it. I feel that I couldn't cut out my exercising completely, but I am a strong-willed person and I feel positive about being able to live with myself if I reduce the intensity gradually. My aim is to keep doing three or four classes of aerobic exercise each week and have the occasional swim. Exercise used to be a really enjoyable feeling for me—now it is an addiction.'

Most women with eating disorders suffering from an exercise disorder talk of 'exercising so they can eat'; in other words, they are usually exercising when they have lower reserves of energy in their body.

Binge-eating disorder

The proposed diagnostic features of binge-eating disorder are described in the box below.

> ## Proposed diagnostic criteria for binge-eating disorder
>
> ◆ The woman has recurrent episodes of binge eating
>
> ◆ She lacks control over her eating during the binge-eating episode
>
> ◆ The binge-eating episodes are associated with at least three of the following: she eats much more rapidly than usual; she eats until she feels uncomfortably full; she eats large amounts of food when not feeling hungry; she eats alone, because she is embarrassed about how much she is eating; she feels disgusted with herself, depressed, or very guilty about overeating
>
> ◆ She is very distressed with regard to her binge eating
>
> ◆ The binge eating occurs, on average, at least 2 days a week for 6 months or more
>
> Modified from the *American Psychiatric Association: Diagnostic and Statistical and Manual of Mental Disorders*, 4th edn (2000), American Psychiatric Association, Washington DC. By permission.

From time to time, many people binge eat (see bulimia nervosa). Usually these people have engaged in periods of dieting or not eaten for many hours before they start binge eating. It is not known why people binge eat and several other reasons have been suggested in addition to a history of episodes of dieting. These include anxiety, depression, and boredom.

 Fact!

10–30% of obese people binge eat.

Women with binge-eating disorder may have suffered previously from anorexia nervosa or bulimia nervosa.

By definition, people with binge-eating disorder do not have anorexia nervosa, as their weight is more than a BMI of 17.5. Neither do they have bulimia nervosa because they do not regularly use dangerous methods of weight control such as starvation, self-induced vomiting, and laxative abuse. Whether a diagnosis of binge-eating disorder should be made, as it is considered somewhat unstable, or whether such patients should be included as part of EDNOS and obesity, has not yet been decided by the American Psychiatric Association. In this book, it is included in both Chapter 9 as a bulimia nervosa-like disorder and in Chapter 11 under obesity and overeating.

Some experts believe that a diagnosis of binge-eating disorder should not be made unless a person is overweight or obese. Currently, we do not know if someone who does not eat during the day and then binge eats at night is any different from a person who does not binge but leads a solitary life so she can be at home by herself in the evening and leisurely eat the food she has bought, knowing that the amount she is consuming will lead to further weight gain.

Obesity

There is controversy among nutritionists as to whether obesity can be classified as an eating disorder. Researchers have shown that obese people choose to eat more food and eat it more quickly than non-obese people. Other researchers have argued that obesity, particularly severe (or morbid) obesity, occurs in people with psychological problems. However, a study of severely obese people in the USA suggested that anxiety, depression, low self-esteem, and poor body image reported by severely obese people were a result, rather than a cause, of their obesity. The experience of nutritionists who try to induce severely obese people to lose weight suggests that obesity is an eating disorder. They report that when severely obese patients are placed on low-energy diets, they have adverse emotional reactions as follows:

◆ 65–75% have a preoccupation with food;

◆ 60–70% become irritable;

◆ 40–50% become nervous; and

◆ 35–45% suffer from depression.

These symptoms are similar to those voiced by bulimic patients and women who have anorexia nervosa. For a few people, there may be a genetic factor that makes it difficult for them to achieve a 'normal' weight (see Chapter 3).

Main features of obesity

High body weight

Obesity can be defined in several ways, some of which require complex investigations and are only practical in research. The simple and effective method is to use the BMI. Inaccuracies can occur for a few muscular men, who do not have sufficient body fat to place them in the obese range but who have a high body weight as muscle weighs more than fat. They can be differentiated from obese people relatively easily.

Two groups can be identified that relate to obesity (Table 2.3). When the person's weight places her in the classification of morbid obesity, medical conditions that are potentially life-threatening become more common and help is required more urgently. Obese, but not overweight, women are also at greater risk of developing medical problems. These groups are arbitrary to some extent.

As for the other eating disorders, there should be no medical or psychiatric illness to account for her high body weight including medications needed in the treatment of these conditions.

Inability to lose body weight

In most cases, it is difficult for an obese person to adhere to a stringent diet, which contains less than 5040 kJ (1200 kcal) per day, because previously she has eaten at least twice and often up to four times this amount of energy each day. She wants to keep to the diet but she is tempted to eat and may binge eat from time to time. The decision to keep to a diet becomes even harder when a severely obese person has already lost substantial weight. Every day, in every

Table 2.3 BMI related to ranges of body weight

Weight group	BMI range (kg/m^2)
Emaciated	Less than 15
Severely underweight	15.0–16.9
Underweight	17.0–18.9
Normal weight range	19.0–24.9
Overweight	25.0–29.9
Obese	30.0–39.9
Severely (morbidly) obese	40.0 or more

social situation, she has to make a decision, and keep to it, that she will not eat food that other people are eating freely. The more she plans to diet, the more she becomes preoccupied with food, and the harder it is for her to keep to her diet.

The main key to weight loss is the motivation to permanently alter eating behaviour, but the obese woman cannot do this, even when confronted with poor health and limited mobility.

Prevalence of eating disorders in the community

 Fact!

Eating disorders can occur among woman of all social classes and racial groups.

The exact prevalence of eating disorders in the community is difficult to determine accurately. Most surveys are made of groups selected for ease of surveying, such as women attending educational institutions. Current information suggests that the figures in Table 2.4 give a reasonable estimate of the prevalence of the eating disorders in the developed world in women aged 15–30.

The prevalence of obesity is more difficult to estimate and it is increasing at different rates in different countries and among different socioeconomic groups. Obesity increases with age and reaches its peak prevalence in both women and men between the ages of 50 and 70.

Table 2.4 Estimation of the prevalence of eating disorders in women in the developed world aged 15–30

Anorexia nervosa	0.5–1.0%
Bulimia nervosa	2% (range 1–3%)
EDNOS*	12% (range 8–23%)
Obesity	10%

*Includes binge-eating disorder.

Future diagnostic criteria

Good diagnostic criteria are needed for eating disorders for best treatment practices and strategies. The criteria given in this chapter are currently being reviewed by the American Psychiatric Association. Until these are available, we find it is useful to describe a person as having an eating disorder and then to refer to the characteristics of the eating disorder that are important for assessment and treatment of an individual person at that time. Patients can have more than one type of eating disorder at the same time and at different times. The types of eating disorder are:

- Low-weight type

- High-weight type

- Vomiting type

- Binge-eating type

- Exercising type

- Atypical, e.g. chewing and spitting.

Or, as we have done in this book, eating disorders can be classified as:

- Anorexia nervosa or anorexia nervosa-like

- Bulimia nervosa or bulimia nervosa-like (can include binge-eating disorder)

- Obesity or overeating disorder (can include binge-eating disorder).

The new criteria are expected to be modified to take into consideration changes in our society as people become more interested in health and fitness rather than body image. Menstrual disturbance will be omitted from the diagnostic criteria because, although it is an excellent measure of the body's reserves of energy, it cannot be determined in women taking oral contraception.

3

Why do eating disorders occur?

Key points

♦ There are theories, but no consensus about why eating disorders occur

♦ A combined explanation of the different 'risk', 'trigger', and 'perpetu-ating' factors contributing to the onset and chronic nature of eating disorders is suggested

♦ The explanations involve genetic, physiological, social, and psycho-logical perspectives and include theories relating to childhood devel-opment and adolescent development

♦ Sexually and physically abused women need more intensive treat-ment and take longer to recover from their eating disorder

'What made me anorexic in the first instance seems to be unimportant compared to what keeps me as thin as I am. I've come to the right conclusion that my anorexia is just a bad habit, and a crutch for any failings I may wish to excuse myself from making.'

In spite of a considerable amount of research over the past three decades, no consensus has been obtained to answer the question of why some adolescents have an eating disorder. Six explanations have been advanced, but none has been proved conclusively. They are: (1) the adolescent development explana-tion; (2) the social explanation; (3) the psychological explanation; (4) the physiological explanation; (5) the genetic explanation; and (6) the childhood developmental explanation. These theories are not mutually exclusive, and referring to more than one may give a closer explanation.

The adolescent development explanation

In our culture, which has an abundance of food, children learn to increase progressively the amount of food they eat, and often increase the quantity of energy they ingest beyond that needed for growth, body functions, and the demands of exercise. In the 3 years before puberty, a biological growth spurt occurs and the food intake is increased further still (see Chapter 1).

The growth spurt in girls occurs between the ages of 12 and 14, and a girl's energy requirements peak over the same period. After her first menstrual period, a girl's energy requirements fall considerably and she gains body fat, as girls do not increase their muscle mass like boys. Most girls consciously or unconsciously reduce their food intake or become more active so that their weight only increases slowly during adolescence. A few girls continue to eat the amount of food they have become accustomed to during the period of growth in early adolescence and put on weight, becoming overweight or obese.

In the year after her first menstrual period, the young woman becomes increasingly aware of her body weight; she begins to learn that she can control weight gain by eating sensibly, changing her eating patterns, dieting, or by using other measures that will help her to stop absorbing the food she eats (see Figures 1.3 and 1.4).

 Patient's perspective

Vera first became concerned about her weight when she was 14, nearly 12 months after her first menstrual period, and she started dieting. However, her preoccupation with food caused her to gain weight, in spite of the diet she had chosen. She was teased about her body by her friends, and in an attempt to lose weight effectively, she began taking large quantities of laxatives when she was 16. Her menstrual periods ceased. The next year, a series of family problems and her continued concern about her body image induced her to adhere to a sensible weight-reducing diet with resultant weight loss. By the age of 18, her weight had stabilized at a level she found acceptable (a body mass index or BMI of 21) and she has maintained this weight, with fluctuations of 1–3 kg (2.2–6.6 lb), for the past 5 years.

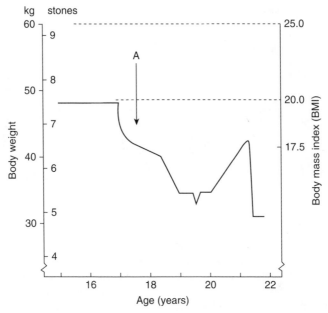

Figure 3.1 Robin started dieting at the age of 14. By the age of 17, she had developed anorexia nervosa (A) and this has persisted in spite of treatment since that date

Some adolescents who diet may become so concerned about control of weight that their eating behaviour escapes from what is considered 'normal' and they develop anorexia nervosa. Those women who respond to dieting by experiencing 'out-of-control' eating episodes (binges) may develop bulimia nervosa or binge-eating disorder. Other women who diet and exercise unsuccessfully or ignore sensible eating information are likely to become obese. A child brought up in an obese family is comfortable with overeating and becoming obese, because she can share an identity with the other members of her family.

Onset of severe weight loss can also follow a period of sensible dieting with realistic weight loss, although in some younger patients it appears to occur suddenly, with no prior unsuccessful or realistic attempts (see Figures 3.1 and 3.2).

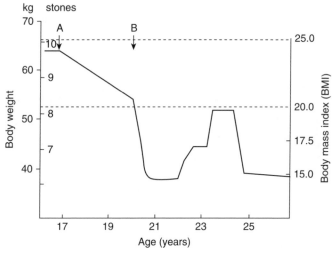

Figure 3.2 Cheryl felt herself to be overweight when she was 17 and started dieting. At that time her BMI was 24 (A). The dieting resulted in a slow weight loss until the age of 20, when she broke up with her boyfriend and had a sudden weight loss, leading to a diagnosis of anorexia nervosa (B)

 Patient's perspective

Kate began to 'watch her weight' when she was at boarding school, as did many of her friends. However, the nature of the food and the supervision of the students limited her ability to control her weight. She left school at 18, having graduated from high school, and became increasingly conscious of her weight. She decided that she wanted to lose weight by 'avoiding eating rubbish'. She was now at university and began binge eating, interspersing this with stringent dieting, which resulted in wide swings in weight. In an attempt to control her weight gain, at the age of 19 she began to self-induce vomiting and abused laxatives. This behaviour coincided with a decision to leave university and to move to another city to take up fashion modelling. To some extent, her behaviour controlled the swings in her weight, but she continued to have episodes of binge eating, although these became less frequent, but it was not until she was 24 that she achieved a body weight below a BMI of 19. She has since stabilized at a BMI of 18.5 by keeping to a strict eating plan, and she no longer uses laxatives.

The social explanation

In Western culture, contrasting messages about food and eating are offered by society, and particularly by the media. The first message is that a slim woman is successful, attractive, healthy, happy, fit, and popular. Most teenagers believe that being slim will help them to be chosen for a good job, find a boyfriend, be popular with their peers, be and look fit and healthy, and get on well with their family (provided that most of the family is not overweight or obese). To become slim, with all that this implies, is deemed to be a major pursuit of many women. The second message is that eating is a pleasurable activity that meets many needs, particularly social contact with friends, in addition to relieving hunger.

Some of the mixed messages from television and women's magazines are:

- You must be slim

- Eating is enjoyable

- Try different foods

- Eat with your friends

- Eat low-energy foods

- Diet

- Eat fast foods

- Do not get fat

- Exercise more.

Families can also give mixed messages. Parents show love and care by providing substantial amounts of food for their children, and their sons and daughters reciprocate by eating it. Yet parents want their children to be healthy and look good. Obese families may encourage weight gain, while the messages at school promote weight loss and more exercise. Not surprisingly, these influences from family, community, and the media provoke conflicting thoughts; a woman can decide to ignore them or to act on some of them. It is not surprising that, in the face of the psychological bombardment of contradictory messages, most young women diet. Some become preoccupied with food and the avoidance of weight gain, developing bulimia or anorexia nervosa. Some decide that dieting is too disturbing to their way of life and return to eating more food than they require, becoming obese.

The psychological explanation

> 'The truth of the matter is that we focus on food and weight so that we don't have to feel any emotions or feelings that may be uncomfortable, such as anger, sadness, anxiety, or guilt.'

Personality

Because eating is such a basic instinct, it has been postulated that those people who suffer from an eating disorder have an identifiable personality. The *Oxford Textbook of Psychiatry* defines personality as '*enduring qualities of an individual shown in his or her ways of behaving in a wide variety of circumstances*'. Studies using personality questionnaires suggest that some women suffering from anorexia nervosa are more 'neurotic', more 'obsessional', more 'self-loathing', and have lower 'self-esteem' than women whose weight is in the 'desirable range'. No distinctive personality profiles are available for women who have bulimia nervosa or for obese women, although most have poor self-esteem. Most women with eating disorders have a 'normal' personality on extensive testing, and the personality scores of normal people and those who suffer from eating disorders overlap considerably.

Personality disorder

The *Oxford Textbook of Psychiatry* defines an abnormal personality as occurring '*when the individual suffers from his own personality or when other people suffer from it*'. The most common characteristics found among patients with eating disorders belong to the 'avoidant/anxious', 'borderline', 'obsessive–compulsive' or 'dependent' types of personality disorder. Few women suffering from an eating disorder will have sufficient of these characteristics for them to receive a diagnosis of a personality disorder, and when these women recover from an eating disorder, only a few have a personality disorder; most do not. Women may have both an eating disorder and a personality disorder, but most people who have an eating disorder do not have a personality disorder.

Patients with bulimia nervosa and patients who induce vomiting are more likely to show features of a 'borderline personality disorder'. For a diagnosis of 'borderline personality disorder' to be made (as defined by The American Psychiatric Association), the person must have at least five of the following eight features: unstable relationships; impulsive behaviour that is harmful to the person (including spending, sex, substance use, shoplifting, reckless driving, and binge eating); variable moods; undue anger or lack of control of anger; recurrent suicidal threats or behaviour; uncertainty about personal identity; persistent feelings of boredom; and frantic efforts to avoid real or imagined abandonment. However, in women with an eating disorder, some of the features can be due to biochemical changes resulting from the eating disorder, e.g. variable moods and anger, while other behaviours can be viewed as 'normal' teenage experimentation and the risk-taking behaviour of their peer group.

Although psychological factors may be involved in explaining why individual patients who have an eating disorder persist with their eating behaviour, no single psychological explanation is available.

The physiological explanation

The control of eating is discussed in Chapter 2. The hormones leptin and ghrenlin are the major messengers modulating the appetite-stimulating neuropeptide Y in the brain. The physiological explanation attempts to relate hormonal changes in appetite and eating with hormonal changes in mood. Research has shown that many people who embark on a strict diet feel 'flat and down in mood'. After eating food, particularly foods with a high carbohydrate content, the level of tryptophan in the blood is raised and crosses from the blood into the brain where it stimulates the production of serotonin (5-hydroxytryptamine, or 5-HT); the raised brain level of serotonin improves the person's mood. Increased leptin levels in the blood going to the brain should also stimulate the release of serotonin and noradrenaline, resulting in feelings of improved mood, satiation, fullness, and a lack of appetite. In other words, if you are hungry, eating makes you feel better and you can relax.

Anorexia nervosa patients initially deny themselves an adequate amount of food and do not respond to the 'messages' to eat more food and feel better. If they continue to eat inadequate amounts of food for their bodily functions over a period of time, one hypothesis suggests that an increase in opioid activity occurs in their brains. This leads to an elevation of the person's mood and causes the person to continue restricting food because it makes them feel 'good'. As time passes, the elevation of mood can only be maintained by reducing the food intake further, and 'addiction' to increased brain opioids may be inevitable if withdrawal symptoms are to be avoided.

Exercise is also thought to cause the release of opioids into the brain, and the more strenuous the exercise, the greater the opioid release. The need for some people to increase the amount of exercise that they undertake can be explained by their need to maintain the release of brain opioids.

Why bulimia nervosa sufferers feel they cannot resist the powerful urge to eat is unknown. It is possible that they become sensitized to one or more of the neuropeptides that drive people to eat, or that they crave feelings of well-being, such as the improved mood and lack of appetite provided by increased brain levels of serotonin after eating. Binge eating may simply arise because the women are constantly dieting to try to attain a body weight that is below their genetically programmed 'weight range', and their physiological response is a normal response to undereating. The conflicting and confusing messages the body receives when bulimics induce vomiting may take many years to be fully understood.

For some reason, obese people appear to be relatively insensitive to leptin. Sufferers of chronic obesity have problems preventing weight gain; most can lose weight but cannot stop it returning. It is likely that leptin is important in this apparent failure of obese people to be able to 'reset' their body weight at a lower weight after weight loss. Genetic influences may explain the insensitivity of the brain to leptin, or the receptors in the brain may adapt and become less affected by high levels of leptin after a long period of time. Some obese people may choose to ignore the feelings of satiation and lack of appetite and continue to eat more food than they require, or they may choose to eat for other reasons including anxiety and sometimes depression.

The genetic explanation

The question of whether a defective gene is the cause of an eating disorder is currently being investigated. There is probably no one gene defect, but rather a combination of genetic factors that increase the likelihood of someone developing an eating disorder. Current studies suggest this could be true in 50–80% of anorexia nervosa and bulimia cases. We know that genes do play a part in the development of anorexia nervosa, bulimia nervosa, eating disorders not otherwise specified (EDNOS), and obesity. These disorders are more common in identical (monozygotic) twins compared with non-identical (dizygotic) twins, and are more common in siblings and families when compared with the general population. Some members of a family develop different eating disorders, e.g. one sister may be bulimic and the other anorexic.

It may be easier to understand the failure to find a defective gene if you consider that people with the genetic potential will only develop an eating disorder if certain events take place, i.e. if events allow the genes to express themselves. A highly respected researcher into the genetics of mental illness, named Kendler, suggests that '*society's current preoccupation with thinness and body image has allowed more people who carry the genes for anorexia nervosa and bulimia nervosa to develop the disorder*'. Fifty years ago, before society emphasized a slim body shape and weight as desirable, these people may not have suffered from an eating disorder as they did not diet. Anything that results in weight loss may allow the 'genes' to show their potential affects.

The same appears to be true for obesity, although an 'obese gene' has been found. This 'obese gene' is thought to induce adipocytes to secrete leptin and possibly explains the apparent insensitivity of some obese people to leptin (see *The physiological explanation* above).

The childhood development explanation

A proportion of patients with eating disorders have had childhood experiences that have an impact on how they respond and cope with events in later life. These can include: the absence of a parent who was ill, bullying at school, family psychiatric illness, or physical or sexual abuse. This explanation suggests that the child does not learn healthy adult ways of coping with situations as she has had no well-functioning role models, and that she has developed unhelpful or destructive ways of coping with some situations and with her moods and feelings.

Physical and sexual abuse

A study of the literature indicates that about 30% of patients with eating disorders will reveal that they were sexually abused in childhood. This incidence of childhood sexual abuse, occurring when the patient was less than 16 years old, is higher than the rate of 10–20% reported among people in the community who have no medical or psychiatric disorder, but is no different to the incidence found among patients suffering from other psychiatric disorders. Abused women usually take longer to respond to treatment for their eating disorder and are more likely to require admission to hospital for treatment.

Women who binge eat or induce vomiting, or both of these, are more likely to have issues with abuse. A study in the USA found that bulimic women were more likely to have experienced sexual abuse as a child than women who suffered from a food-restricting disorder. Sexual abuse as an older adolescent or adult would also be expected to be more common among bulimic eating-disorder women as they are more sexually active and more 'at risk' because of their sexual behaviour.

Patient's perspective

Catriona vividly described her experiences of abuse and its association with food as a child and her difficulties as an adult not only with anxiety and her eating-disordered behaviour, but in relating to men. She is now a successful lawyer with two children.

'I recount the following events of my childhood and the ongoing results that those events have had on my life: anxiety and an atypical eating disorder. I can recall my father would leave home early in the morning and return home at night, usually drunk, and often angry, which generally led to violent verbal and physical arguments. Dad would usually arrive home around the time of the evening meal. Mum had been trying to coax my sister into eating something from her plate. She was a poor eater and there was a constant argument between my mother and sister during meal times. I was always praised for eating everything put in front of me. I wanted to be a "good" daughter for my mother, because I believed it would make her life happier.

During meal times, I recall being incredibly anxious waiting for my father to knock on the front door. If the knock was loud and hard, then we knew he would be angry. I would then move into control mode. I would take charge of the situation, always telling my mother not to say anything that might provoke my father's anger. I felt a tremendous burden of having to control my father's violence and anger. I would always put myself between Mum and my sister when he would threaten them, both physically and verbally. I would talk quietly and calmly; sometimes it would calm him, other times it would not. He would go into a rage and then start hitting Mum. On these occasions, we would usually have to leave the house and run to the next-door neighbours. I can recall the police being called. My mother suffered numerous injuries during our childhood—a broken nose, broken fingers, as well as other injuries such as bruised legs, bruised arms, etc. Dad would deny that he had done anything the next morning.

When I was successful in calming him, he would go into the lounge room to eat his dinner. I can recall how revolting it was to watch him eat. He would either drop food on his clothes or dribble down the side of his mouth. I used to cringe as I had to sit with him, feeling revolted by the whole picture. I used to think he was a dirty pig. When he had finished, Dad would call me to sit with him while he watched TV. I can recall feeling forced to sit with him in the lounge, with his arm around me, until he fell asleep. I would then very gently remove his arm and leave.

Dad would sometimes not return home before we went to bed. I used to lie awake on these nights waiting until he came home. I suffered from shocking nightmares . . .

As an adult, I found it incredible difficulty knowing how to relate to men without giving them the wrong signals. I always tried to be friendly to avoid any potentially aggressive situations. However, on reflection, this friendliness that I used to protect myself often became a cause for unwanted advances, which I felt I had no skills to handle. I used to feel so upset because I knew I should be able to deal with the situations as an adult, and yet I felt like a child in a woman's body, unable to speak up.'

The combined explanation

No single explanation is sufficient to explain why eating disorders occur. What we do know is that many factors are involved. One common initiating feature of anorexia nervosa, bulimia nervosa, binge-eating disorder, and possibly obesity is weight loss or attempted weight loss. In other words, when the body's energy balance is disturbed, the body reacts to counteract this upset. A flow chart of risk factors, trigger factors, and perpetuating factors is shown in Figure 3.3.

Trigger factors

The triggers for the initial weight loss or continued attempts at weight loss can occur for many reasons. Common reasons cited by teenagers are a viral illness, stress due to life events such as losing a parent, depression, stress at school with examinations or friends, going overseas, increasing exercise to improve performance for a forthcoming sporting competition, joining a gym, and of course trying to change your body image.

Risk factors

We have already considered some of the risk factors, including a genetic propensity to develop an eating disorder. Other, possibly genetically determined, candidates may be: tolerance of weight loss or gain; impulse control around food; 'picky' food habits even as a child; ease of inducing vomiting; and failure of compensatory mechanisms for overeating or undereating, including lack of an accurate perception of feeling full or empty. As we have seen, being female and first menstruation (menarche) are also predisposing factors.

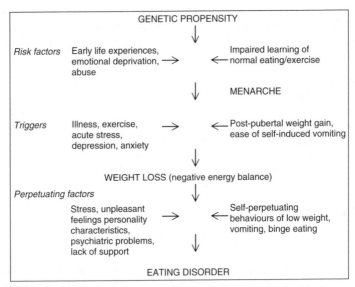

Figure 3.3 Risk factors, trigger factors, and perpetuating factors involved in the development and maintenance of eating disorders

Early childhood factors can play a part, particularly if the normal parent–child interactions are interrupted, as is the case if one parent is ill and away in hospital, if another sibling is chronically ill and needs a lot of parental care, if a parent is an alcoholic or drug abuser, or if the parents are distant and uncaring. These early experiences can impair the psychological development of the person, and in some of these cases a failure to learn normal eating patterns occurs. In others, there may also be unusual emphasis placed on food and the significance of food and eating in the family—as compensation, restriction, or to show disapproval (see *Patient's perspective*: Catriona, above).

Perpetuating factors

The perpetuating factors are usually multiple and different for everyone, and include the advantages an eating disorder provides (page 78). These range from 'keeping parents talking to each other' to blocking out unpleasant emotions and avoiding adolescent and adult challenges.

There are other maintaining aspects of eating disorder behaviour that may have a biological and genetic basis, that is, once the behaviours have commenced they are self-perpetuating. Being at a low weight can be continued so that some people cannot gain weight without considerable help. This is seen when a certain breed of rat is put in a running cage, and as long as it is well fed, the rat will run until it is tired, when it will stop and rest; if you starve one of these rats before putting it in a running cage, it will keep running until it collapses and dies. It is believed that changes in the brain chemicals of the starved rat drive it to keep active and keep moving to find food. When patients are recovered, they can talk about knowing that there is a weight they cannot go below, because if they do they will fall into the weight-losing spiral again. Binge eating interspersed with attempts to lose weight is also self-perpetuating, usually leading to obesity and, most addictive of all, self-induced vomiting. Preliminary evidence suggests that people who 'genetically' find it easy to induce vomiting may be more likely to develop a chronic eating disorder. In all of these cases, it is likely that we will understand these behaviours much better when we know more about the neuropeptide neurotransmitter substances of the brain and about the appetite and feeding hormones involved in the energy balance of the body when these behaviours are present.

'Most anorexics do not set out with the aim of losing weight to any extent. However, once it has begun, it is extremely difficult to control. Then you need help in order to stop the destructive pattern and to regain some normality in your life.'

4

Infertility, pregnancy, and the postpartum period

> ## ➜ Key points
>
> ◆ Women with eating and exercise disorders may have difficulty falling pregnant; small improvements in their behaviour or weight can assist their fertility
>
> ◆ Women who are underweight at the time of conception or who do not gain enough weight during pregnancy have a greater risk of restricting the growth of their baby
>
> ◆ Women suffering from bulimia nervosa are at greater risk of miscarrying, having their baby die just before birth, or having the baby born prematurely
>
> ◆ Obese women are more likely to have difficulties during childbirth and are at higher risk of developing gestational diabetes mellitus and pregnancy-induced hypertension
>
> ◆ Women with a history of an eating disorder are more likely to experience mood disturbances during pregnancy and postnatal depression
>
> ◆ It is not possible to predict whether a woman who is recovering from an eating disorder will relapse or will be free from her problem during her pregnancy

Body image challenge

Pregnancy is a major challenge to a woman's body weight and body image. During pregnancy, changes take place slowly at first and then quite quickly as the pregnancy progresses (Figure 4.1). The first noticeable change

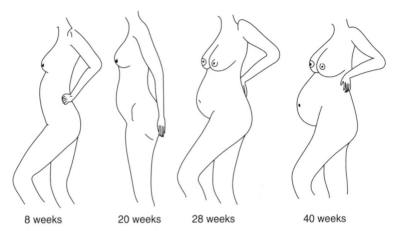

| 8 weeks | 20 weeks | 28 weeks | 40 weeks |

Figure 4.1 Body image changes during pregnancy

is an increase in the size of the breasts. These are like the premenstrual chang-es of fullness and tenderness familiar to many women, but during pregnancy the breasts continue to enlarge. Some women with small breasts may be delighted with these changes, while women who worry about the large size of their breasts may find these changes uncomfortable and may feel self-conscious about their body image.

From very early in pregnancy, changes in hormones, produced by the placenta, prepare the body for the needs of the developing fetus. In early preg-nancy, the mother easily supplies the oxygen and nutrients for her developing fetus and can continue moderate amounts of low-intensity exercise. As the demands made by the fetus increase, the mother slows down her activities and body functioning. At this stage of pregnancy, most women exercise very lightly, if at all, feel relaxed, and do not feel like doing very much. This allows energy to be stored in the form of fat in the breasts, hips, and thighs. This 'passivity' of pregnancy is essential for the growth and development of the baby, but has a few disadvantages for mothers: two of these are constipation due to decreased motility of the gut and excess weight gain if she does not eat a sensible diet.

Weight gain during pregnancy

Weight gain during pregnancy is necessary. Until recently, it was believed that the baby would derive all the energy and nutrition it required from its mother, even

Table 4.1 Factors contributing to weight gain during pregnancy

Reasons for weight gain during pregnancy	Approximate weight gain during pregnancy (%)
Fetus and placenta	32
Breasts and uterus	10
Increase in blood volume	10
Fat deposited	22
Water retained	26

if the mother was in a state of starvation. There is now evidence to show that women who maintain low body weights and women who restrict their weight gain during pregnancy are more likely to give birth to a growth-retarded baby.

To understand weight gain during pregnancy, it can be helpful to examine what contributes to the weight gain. The increased size of the breasts, the fetus and amniotic fluid that protects the fetus, the placenta that transports the oxygen and nutrients from mother to fetus and takes away the waste products, and the deposition of fat on the breasts, thighs, and hips are obvious contributors. Less obvious is the 6–8 litres of fluid that are added to the body of the mother. Water is retained due to the action of the pregnancy hormones on the tissues of the body. Additional fluid is needed to make up the large increase in blood volume that is necessary to carry oxygen and nutrients to the growing fetus. The approximate contributions of these factors to the overall weight gain of a woman of average weight and height during pregnancy are given in Table 4.1. The actual amounts are highly variable, as every woman is different and every baby is different.

 Fact!

Most of the weight gain during pregnancy is fluid, baby, and placenta.

Deposition of fat on the tissues of the breasts, hips, and thighs is under the influence of the pregnancy hormones. This store of energy ensures that the woman is able to continue to provide for her baby after the birth by being able to feed and take care of her baby. The media often only show photographs of glamorous, scantily clad, or naked pregnant women that obscure this normal shape or are changed by computer to have the fat distribution of a non-pregnant woman.

> **Fact!**
>
> The deposition and distribution of fat on the breasts, hips, and thighs is a normal part of pregnancy.

Weight gain is more rapid after about 20 weeks of pregnancy. An 'average' woman who does not restrict her food intake or act in a way that allows her to maintain a body weight below her normal weight can expect to gain about 3 kg (7 lb) in the first 20 weeks and about 9 or 10 kg (20 lb) in the second 20 weeks. Many women, if they are weighed during pregnancy, will find their weight varies widely and they do not follow the pattern suggested above. Most women gain 10–15 kg, on average 12.5 kg (22–33 lb, on average 27 lb), during pregnancy.

The amount of weight a mother needs to gain in pregnancy will vary. Underweight women need to gain an amount of weight to give them a body weight before pregnancy in the normal weight range (body mass index (BMI) of 19–25) as well as the normal healthy weight gain expected during pregnancy. If an underweight mother tries to restrict her weight gain, particularly in early pregnancy, she may be failing to provide her infant with optimal growth and development in the uterus. Overweight and obese women do not need to put on as much weight during pregnancy, probably because they already have reserves of energy to ensure the development of their future infant.

Eating during pregnancy

Most pregnant women will find that they are eating slightly more, perhaps an extra glass of milk and an extra two slices of bread each day. The idea of 'eating for two' is incorrect and will lead to increases in the amount of fat being stored in the body in excess of the amount required for a healthy pregnancy. A woman who 'eats for two' will not be able to lose this excess weight and return to her pre-pregnancy weight in the year after her baby is born. Many women report that their eating and nutrition improves during pregnancy— they eat more regularly and eat more nutritious foods that they understand will help their baby thrive. About 20% of women feel their eating deteriorates, usually in response to concerns about the amount of weight they are gaining. This may occur because women are weighed during their antenatal visits and then told how much weight they have gained.

Other women may commence binge eating when they try to adhere to the advice of some doctors who mistakenly believe weight gain during pregnancy should be 'as little as possible'.

Binge eating and food cravings

Binge eating can occur during pregnancy and for 7% of women who have never suffered from an eating disorder, this may be the first time they have experienced disordered eating. This is the time when the fetus is growing rapidly and making increasing demands on the mother for food. Women who have ignored the messages to eat more to supply the demands of their baby, either because they were occupied with other aspects of their busy life or because they were trying to prevent gaining 'too much weight', are likely to eat quickly and to continue to eat once they start eating. This resembles binge eating. Eating in response to this inadequate maternal food intake may explain some of the binge eating of pregnancy. Binge eating may also follow the nausea and vomiting of early pregnancy if, because of vomiting, insufficient energy has been available for storage in the mother's body.

 Fact!

Binge eating is more common in the second half of pregnancy.

Other triggers for binge eating may be boredom associated with decreased activity, worry about the future, and preoccupation with thoughts of food. Craving for certain foods is common during pregnancy. These cravings are very diverse and vary from woman to woman. The foods may have a high water content, such as watermelon and oranges, or be high in fat and carbohydrate, such as pizza and Mexican food, or high in carbohydrates, such as bananas. The foods craved may taste spicy, bland, bitter, or salty. It is thought that these cravings reflect the needs of the woman's body and that eating these foods, in moderation, will provide her with the nutrients she is lacking.

Contraception

Women with anorexia nervosa or bulimia nervosa may have been prescribed oral contraceptives for contraception or for hormone replacement to prevent further loss of bone density. Women taking 'the pill' as prescribed, unless they are very emaciated, will experience a 'withdrawal bleed'. This menstrual-like bleeding occurs because the 'pill' hormones are stopped or 'withdrawn' for 7 of the 28 days of the 'pill' cycle.

Fact!

You will not know if you will have amenorrhoea if you are taking oral contraception.

The occurrence of a 'withdrawal bleed' does not mean that menstruation and a normal ovulatory menstrual cycle will occur when 'the pill' is ceased. Women who commence oral contraception when they are having regular menses and then develop an eating disorder may find that they are amenorrhoeic (no periods) when they stop 'the pill'. If women recover from their eating disorder before stopping oral contraception, menstruation is likely to occur.

Getting pregnant

Both underweight and overweight women, and women with eating and exercise disorders, may have difficulties falling pregnant. Women who desire fertility should be encouraged to accept help with their disordered eating before becoming pregnant. It may not be possible to achieve a 'cure' for the eating disorder before they wish to conceive, but small changes in behaviour can help conception. When underweight women begin to increase their body weight and obese women lose some weight, the levels of hormones involved in reproduction improve and ovulation can occur. Decreasing the frequency or ceasing methods of weight loss that are stressful to the body also improves the chances of pregnancy. Learning to eat regularly throughout the day and exercising sensibly may be sufficient for normal-weight women who are recovering from their eating disorder to conceive.

 Fact!

Treatment of disordered eating can prevent the need for assisted conception.

However, if an eating-disorder sufferer, in conjunction with her partner, feels that recovery from her eating disorder will take too long or will not be successful, they can be reassured that 'assisted conception', although expensive and uncomfortable, is usually successful. Treatment with hormones used to induce ovulation, IVF (*in vitro* fertilization), or one of the newer technologies will usually result in pregnancy. Unfortunately, these methods of assisted conception are more likely to result in miscarriage and several attempts may be needed. There are also risks with the treatment. Drugs used to induce ovulation may cause excessive ovarian enlargement (ovarian hypersensitivity syndrome), which in some cases leads to abdominal pain, fluid in the abdomen, a fall in blood pressure, and in a few cases life-threatening blood coagulation changes. These changes are reversible for the majority of women.

Eating disorders and management during pregnancy

Women suffering from disordered eating are more likely to experience complications during their pregnancy and after the birth. Complications during pregnancy include:

* an increased risk of miscarriage;

* vomiting that requires treatment in hospital (hyperemesis gravidarum);

* pregnancy-induced hypertension;

* gestational diabetes;

* delivery of a small growth-retarded baby;

* delivery of a premature baby;

* delivery of a large baby.

Complications after birth (postpartum) include:

* postpartum haemorrhage;

* postnatal depression;

* feelings of distress.

There is accumulating evidence being published in scientific journals to suggest that the uterine environment in which babies develop and grow may affect their quality of life as an adult. This warm, protective, and nurturing environment is influenced by maternal behaviours including her eating, drinking, and exercise.

To ensure that women with eating disorders give their babies the best possible start in life, nutritional, psychological, and medical support must be available during their pregnancies. Each woman should be assessed by members of a multidisciplinary team early in pregnancy and introduced to people who can help her if she needs information or finds that her eating becomes a problem later in pregnancy. Most treatment will consist of reassurance, particularly about weight and shape issues and pregnancy symptoms, and support both during and after the birth. To help women suffering from eating disorders, some suggestions have been made for health professionals to improve the quality of antenatal and postnatal care; these are shown in the box below. The woman's partner or family should be included in the assessment and they should also be offered support during pregnancy and after childbirth.

Suggestions for health professionals for the antenatal care of women with eating disorders

1. *Pre-pregnancy body weight.* Ask about the weight immediately before pregnancy and calculate the woman's BMI. If above 30 or below 18, the woman should be assessed very carefully and followed more intensely during pregnancy.

2. *Measure height.* The height given by women is not always accurate.

3. *Measure body weight during some visits.* Explain to each woman that you need to know her body weight during pregnancy, as this is one piece of information that tells you her baby is growing normally. Body weight is no longer measured routinely in many antenatal clinics, as women often do not like to be weighed.

4. *Ask women if they want to be told their body weight.* Some pregnant women (10–20%), particularly if they have an eating disorder, will become more preoccupied with thoughts of food and will experience deterioration in their eating behaviour if they are told their weight. These women can be weighed with their back turned towards the scales.

5. *Assess nutrition, eating, and weight-controlling behaviour.* A person who is experienced with nutrition during pregnancy and eating disorders should make this assessment. This assessment should be made as early in pregnancy as possible and again early in the third trimester. 'At risk' women should be followed throughout pregnancy and for the first year after the birth.

6. *Assess exercise behaviour and lifestyle.* This assessment should examine the type and amount of exercise, including walking, which may not be considered part of an exercise programme.

---

7. *Medications being taken.* Most women try to avoid taking any medications when they are pregnant. Women with disordered eating patterns are more likely to smoke cigarettes for weight control and to take antidepressant medication.

8. *Nausea and vomiting.* Hyperemesis gravidarum is more common in women with eating disorders during pregnancy. Women with and without eating disorders admit to vomiting during pregnancy to feel better and to prevent weight gain. Most women are able to decrease their frequency of vomiting when they know it may affect their baby.

9. *Provide information about eating and body weight.* Information needs to be provided to women during and after each pregnancy. Most women are concerned about weight gain and weight loss changes in body shape and the effect of changing their eating and exercise behaviour. Woman's experiences and concerns change during pregnancy, during breastfeeding, and during her adaptation to motherhood.

10. *Assess prenatal and postnatal moods.* Women with a history of an eating disorder are more likely to experience mood disturbances and postnatal depression. The depressed mood may be present before, during, and after pregnancy and may not occur until 3 or 6 months after the birth.

11. *Breastfeeding.* Women may breastfeed because they believe this will aid weight loss after pregnancy. Women need to eat more while they are breastfeeding and to adjust their eating patterns again after ceasing breastfeeding.

12. *Previous psychiatric history.* A previous history of psychological or psychiatric problems should be sought, particularly of depression, alcohol dependence, and eating disorders. Women with a previous history should be treated as 'at risk' during and for 12 months after pregnancy.

High- and low-birthweight babies

Women suffering from eating disorders during pregnancy are more likely to have babies that are smaller or larger than 90% of babies born. Small babies and large babies are more likely to have health problems in childhood and as adults. Babies who are of low body weight when they are born may be growth-retarded *in utero* or preterm. A growth-retarded baby is small for the number of weeks of pregnancy when it is born (or during pregnancy when it is measured during ultrasound examination), while a preterm baby is small because it is born too early (less than 37 weeks of pregnancy). Babies can be both growth-retarded and preterm.

Fact!

Growth restriction during pregnancy is associated with hypertension, insulin resistance, diabetes, and cardiovascular disease as an adult.

There is now overwhelming evidence from both Western and Asian countries that people who were small at birth because they failed to grow, rather than because they were born too early, have a greater risk of coronary heart disease, stroke, hypertension, and type 2 diabetes. They are also more likely to develop metabolic syndrome or insulin resistance syndrome. These findings are independent of the person's BMI, smoking and alcohol habits, activity and social class. This effect of growth restriction *in utero* has been confirmed in twin studies, and some of these changes have already occurred by puberty.

Glucose is the main source of energy needed for the body's cells to function. Insulin is a hormone produced by the pancreas that helps cells take in glucose and convert it to energy in the cells, particularly in the liver and muscles where any excess can also be stored as glycogen until it is needed. If there is insulin resistance or not enough insulin produced, glucose cannot be taken into the cells and it will build up in the blood stream.

It is hypothesized that if insufficient glucose is available for the baby when it should be growing in the uterus, then the production of insulin will be low and any glucose that is available will be used by the vital organs (heart) and not for growth. The growth factor responsible for fetal growth, which is very like insulin in structure (called insulin-like growth factor), will be switched off, leading to growth retardation. During childhood, if food is plentiful, there can be a fast 'catch-up' in growth as the growth factors and insulin are stimulated, but insulin resistance develops. It is not fully understood why this occurs, but the impairment *in utero* and changes in the insulin-like growth factors are implicated. This insulin resistance means that an adult is more likely to become obese, diabetic, and hypertensive. A study in the UK found that adolescent girls who were smallest at birth and 'fattest' at the age of 14–16 appeared to be programmed by their restricted growth during fetal life and 'catch-up growth' during childhood to store their fat centrally on the trunk of their body rather than on their arms and legs. Central obesity is a risk factor for many health problems.

Intrauterine growth-restricted infants born to mothers of low body weight are reported to be at increased risk of cognitive disorders including the development of attention-deficit hyperactive disorder or ADHD.

Large babies are also more likely to be overweight as children and adults. In a recent study of Portuguese children, the most important risk factors found for being overweight and obese in childhood were having overweight parents or being of high birthweight. In this Portuguese study, the researchers found that educating parents about obesity was protective and helped to prevent the development of obesity in these 'at risk' children.

Anorexia nervosa and pregnancy

Pregnancy, particularly if unexpected, may pose several challenges to women who are recovering or have recovered from anorexia nervosa. Some women look forward to the pregnancy, feeling that during pregnancy and when caring for a child they will be less preoccupied with body weight and eating, and that 'pregnant women are allowed to be fat'. These women find being pregnant provides relief from their eating and weight-losing behaviours. Other women may become extremely distressed and anxious with the changes in their body image and report an exacerbation or no change in their eating-disordered behaviours.

The desire to become pregnant can be sufficiently strong to induce some women to increase their weight and try to recover from anorexia nervosa or to increase their weight to achieve ovulation and pregnancy, even if they return to a low weight between each pregnancy (see *Patient's perspective*: Anna). Other women prefer to have ovulation induced and accept assisted conception (see *Getting pregnant*, above). During pregnancy, anorexia nervosa sufferers may become distressed and feel that they cannot put on weight. They may accept this and lose weight or allow themselves to gain a small amount of weight that they feel will be lost easily after the birth. Other women enjoy their pregnancy and gain the amount of weight necessary to ensure delivering a baby who has achieved its full growth potential before the birth.

 Patient's perspective

Anna had a 12-year history of anorexia nervosa and excessive exercise before her first baby. She has five children and has had three miscarriages. Ovulation induction was not successful and resulted in either no pregnancy or pregnancy loss (twins and two other singleton babies). All of her living children were conceived naturally: three were conceived 1 or 2 months after a miscarriage. The births were all relatively uneventful; three babies were born spontaneously at 38–40 weeks of gestation and two were born after labour was induced at 42 weeks. Her babies' birthweights were all in the normal range. Anna had no postpartum depression and enjoys her role as a mother; she works part-time and she and her husband share the childcare. All of the children are well and thriving. After three girls and two boys, she feels her family is complete. She wrote the following about her experiences:

'To view it from the outside looks like it was very simple to achieve five children—quite the contrary. It has been a real struggle to gain the weight to conceive a family. Infertility drugs certainly helped me to gain weight in order to conceive. It appears that if my weight fell slightly during pregnancy, I miscarried or threatened to miscarry. I think with my first miscarriage I had felt very responsible and guilty, as it was probably my eating disorder that had caused the problem. It seems the first trimester is the most problematic as it requires my hormones to support the baby and those hormone levels were probably at a minimum. If I made it into the second trimester, I carried through to term. I decided if I was going to be pregnant, I did not want to restrict/starve to prevent problems with the baby. I decided to put my eating disorder into remission for 9 months. I created a "pregnant self". This "pregnant self" had a new lot of rules that needed to be abided to for 9 months: no excessive exercise, no starving or restricting, follow a normal eating plan suitable for pregnancy and to gain the 10–12 kg necessary in pregnancy.

When I looked in a mirror and gained weight it was not "fat"; it became "I'm pregnant". I was able to stick to these rules every day of pregnancy. It was like I flicked on a "pregnancy switch". As a reward, I allowed myself after the pregnancy to lose the weight with restriction but not lower than 950–1000 calories a day. Breastfeeding was difficult because as soon as I started to restrict, it was difficult to feed and I would have unsettled babies and would move them to bottles. I would not let my weight drop below 64 kg as I knew it would be difficult to conceive again. If I wanted to conceive again, I would have to gain another 2 kg to fall pregnant and not miscarry. I seemed to have fewer problems at 66–68 kg.

Overall, I was able to gain the weight as I had the motivation of wanting a baby. Having had one and realizing it was not going to be as devastating as I thought, I certainly knew what I needed to be able to do to have more.'

Recently, we studied healthy women who had delivered their first baby in the previous week. We found that 32% of women who gave birth to a growth-retarded baby were suffering from an eating disorder, usually anorexia nervosa or an eating or exercise disorder involving low body weight. The mothers who were most 'at risk' of retarding the growth and development of their babies in the uterus were:

- those with a low BMI (<19) before pregnancy and at the time of conception;

- those who failed to gain adequate weight during pregnancy;

- those who reported they were overeating during the pregnancy when they must have been undereating;

- those who were more likely to have an eating disorder.

To avoid growth retardation of her baby, a woman who is underweight should be helped to increase her body weight early in pregnancy. The woman may need help from a dietician and reassurance from her physician to achieve an appropriate weight gain. This will include the weight she needed to gain before pregnancy to be at a pre-pregnancy weight in the normal body weight range (BMI >19) plus the normal healthy weight gain expected during a pregnancy.

Intrauterine growth retardation is also associated with smoking cigarettes. Many women smoke cigarettes to help control their body weight and maintain lower body weights, and 4% continue to smoke during pregnancy to control their weight. Women who smoke and who have a low body weight need extra care during pregnancy, from both their physician and their dietician.

Bulimia nervosa and pregnancy

Women with bulimia nervosa can respond to pregnancy in various ways. Some may cease binge eating and self-induced vomiting 'to protect their baby' or they may find that these behaviours stop because they become relaxed about their body shape and weight and feel that pregnancy provides 'an excuse not to look perfect'. Other women report that their eating disorder becomes worse, usually in the last third of pregnancy, when they begin to worry about losing weight after the birth. If women are binge eating and purging every day before pregnancy, these behaviours can continue unchanged throughout pregnancy and the postnatal period (see *Patient's perspective*: Anthea).

Patient's perspective

Anthea had gained very little weight during her first pregnancy. In her second pregnancy, she was repeating this pattern and sought help. After discharge from the Eating Disorders Unit, she wrote:

'What a battle it's been trying to gain weight so that I can have a healthy baby and at the same time still have the desire to keep my weight down. As you know, I tried hard on my own but didn't have much success. After 10 years of having an eating disorder, the fact that I was carrying a child was not enough for me to stop my behaviour. I kept thinking back to my first pregnancy—no morning sickness, healthy and fit the whole way through, and I gave birth to a perfectly healthy and beautiful baby girl—knowing that my weight gain and eating habits throughout that pregnancy were far from normal. But I was anxious the whole time that my lack of weight gain would harm the baby.

I knew that I couldn't take the same risks again and so spent 8 weeks at the Unit. The time I spent there was more than helpful, although the separation from my baby and husband was more difficult than I had ever imagined. My weight gain in hospital was quite considerable initially and quite difficult to come to terms with, so I had to keep remembering exactly why I was there: the sooner I came to terms with that, the sooner I'd be back at home with my family.

My first week home was quite difficult, the hardest thing being the rejection from my daughter. Daddy was her hero and I'd taken the back seat. Feeling very sorry for myself, I found myself quite depressed and very tempted to return to my former eating habits. I must admit that I had some difficult moments but I managed to fight these bad times.

After being home now for 6 weeks and with about 10 weeks to go, I feel so proud to be pregnant! I know that my weight gain has slowed down, but my eating habits are a lot more normal than in my first pregnancy, which makes me very content and very ready for the birth of another baby.

The thing for me to remember is that, after I've had this baby, my body isn't going to return to normal straight away. At this stage, I don't know how I will react, but I will face it when the time comes.'

Women who vomit a lot during the first 12–16 weeks of pregnancy or who induce vomiting during pregnancy have a greater chance of delivering a lower-birthweight baby. These babies are more likely to be born early rather than being growth-retarded at birth. Bulimia nervosa sufferers are more likely to:

◆ miscarry (spontaneously abort their fetus in the first half of pregnancy);

◆ have a preterm baby (born early but at normal weight for number of weeks of pregnancy); or

◆ have a baby die just before or after the birth.

Certainly women suffering from bulimia nervosa are more likely to experience an unwanted pregnancy and are more likely to seek to terminate their pregnancy than women who do not have an eating disorder.

Some bulimic women vomit more than their pregnancy would explain: they allow themselves to vomit in response to the nausea experienced by pregnant women 'to feel better', 'to get rid of the nausea', and to 'avoid weight gain'. A few women may need to be treated for their vomiting in hospital (hyperemesis gravidarum). Whether women who have trained themselves to vomit easily after eating are more likely to have difficulties stopping vomiting during pregnancy is unknown.

Obesity and pregnancy

Overweight and obese women do not all have eating disorders, but a proportion binge eat and may increase their weight excessively in pregnancy. Excess weight gain, i.e. greater than 16 kg during pregnancy, is difficult to lose in the year following the birth unless the woman is able to follow a strict menu plan and to exercise. Natural weight loss after pregnancy is thought to be under genetic control so, if this is true, some women who have gained less than 15 kg will also be unable to lose this weight without exercise and a reduced energy intake.

 Fact!

A small weight loss by obese women in preparation for pregnancy can reduce the incidence of medical complications.

Obese women also respond to pregnancy in different ways. Some women can start eating regularly and sensibly 'for their baby', even if they cannot do it at other times. Other women who are good at dieting for months at a time but unable to limit their intake when they are not dieting can frequently employ 'sensible eating' as a 'diet' during pregnancy. Other obese women continue their behaviours, overeat, and feel out of control.

Women who are obese at the onset of pregnancy may require additional antenatal care, as they are more likely to develop complications during pregnancy including:

* gestation diabetes mellitus;

* pregnancy-induced hypertension.

Pregnancy-induced hypertension is diagnosed when a woman's blood pressure increases above 140 (systolic) and 90 (diastolic). Her blood pressure must be treated to prevent eclampsia (convulsions and coma) developing. It may be necessary to deliver her baby early, by caesarean section, if her blood pressure cannot be reduced.

Maternal obesity is associated with other difficulties in labour leading to caesarean section, postpartum haemorrhage, and a poorer outcome of pregnancy. Morbidly obese women, and women who suffer from pre-gestational and gestation diabetes deliver babies that are large for gestational age (LGA). To reduce the risk of the birth of an LGA infant, it is recommended that maternal weight gain during pregnancy should not exceed 12 kg or 25 lbs.

Obese women who deliver their first child are more likely to deliver a very preterm infant (less than 31 weeks of gestation) and have an increased risk of their fetus dying late in pregnancy. Poor weight gain during pregnancy may be associated with an increased risk of low-birthweight and growth-retarded babies to mothers who are obese. For this reason, women who elect to have weight-reduction operations are advised to use very safe methods of contraception during the rapid weight loss that follows the surgery. This is particularly important for those women who have failed to conceive because of their obesity, as fertility may increase following even a small loss of weight.

Past sufferers of eating disorders

During pregnancy, women who have recovered from their eating disorder are similar to women who have never had disordered eating. They are not more likely to miscarry, lose their babies later in pregnancy, experience complications during pregnancy and the postnatal period, or deliver large, preterm, or small babies.

Fact!

Women with a past history of an eating disorder may experience some disordered thoughts, fears, and preoccupation with food and body weight during pregnancy.

It is not possible to predict whether a woman who is recovering from disordered eating and exercise will be free from her problems during pregnancy. She may experience an improvement, an exacerbation, a relapse, or report no change in her eating or exercise. One woman can respond in a different way during and after each of her pregnancies.

Postnatal distress and postnatal depression

Women suffering from anorexia nervosa and bulimia nervosa are more likely to seek help for distress and depression in the year after the birth of a child, particularly if it is their first child. In a recent study, we found that women who are most at risk of postnatal mood problems are more likely to use dangerous methods of weight control, such as self-induced vomiting, or to binge eat.

Women give a range of explanations for their postnatal problems. Many have unrealistic and idealized expectations of motherhood, mistakenly believing that having a child will solve their problems by giving them something to think about (apart from themselves), making their partner more loving, or giving them someone to love. Some wanted to 'feel more like a woman' or be accepted by their families. Many women have no partner or supports.

Many women do not realize what hard work it is to take care of a baby. Women who are depressed during pregnancy can remain depressed after pregnancy, and women with a previous history of depression are more likely to become depressed in the few years after the birth of a child. Postpartum depression is thought to result from the changes in hormones in a woman's body after giving birth, which affect the neurotransmitter chemicals in the brain that influence mood.

Women suffering from eating disorders need additional support during the postnatal period. Time away from her infant, reassurance that she is coping well, practical information, and help coping with her child will decrease her distress. Mild exercise can help prevent depressed moods following childbirth, but for some women it may be suggested that they take antidepressant medication.

Breastfeeding

Currently, women believe that weight loss will be quicker if they breastfeed, so most women who are conscious of their body weight and shape breastfeed their baby.

 Fact!

A breastfeeding woman requires more energy (in the form of food) than during pregnancy.

For her body to obtain this energy, she receives messages from the brain that tell her to eat more food and drink more fluid. Most women will find it extremely difficult to restrict their food intake at this time, as they will experience constant thoughts of food and feel the need to eat and drink if they do try to limit their intake. Some women find difficulty decreasing the amount of food eaten in the few weeks after lactation has stopped, while some women binge eat in response to trying to not eat.

If women are not coping well because of fatigue and they are feeling down in their mood and not enjoying breastfeeding, they can be reassured and given permission to cease breastfeeding. In a study of women without eating disorders, we found that immediately after ceasing breastfeeding women felt that their mood improved, they were less fatigued, and they were more interested in sexual matters. Women also associate the progesterone-only 'pill' (taken for contraception between pregnancies) with a depressed mood.

Parenthood

Women's concerns about their eating behaviour and attitudes to body weight may interfere with their care of the child. The woman may be overly concerned about her child's weight and shape and this may affect the child's eating behaviour. Women who are trying to teach their children 'good eating habits' and prevent them from becoming 'overweight' may restrict the type and amount of food they give their children. These children may be hungry and feel different from their friends and they may steal food from other children's lunch boxes. Other women fear that their judgement of normal eating may be inaccurate and become overconcerned that they may deprive their children of food so may inadvertently overfeed their infant.

Fact!

The majority of women with a history of disordered eating respond well to their role as a mother and find it a very positive experience.

Children become aware of mothers who do not eat with the family, who only eat once or twice a day, or who graze throughout the day. Children learn by example. Patients have reported pre-school children asking why their mother goes to the bathroom after dinner or why she only eats in the kitchen and not with them.

'It is all coming together, gradually. I just hope that I am not going to do too much damage to my kids whilst I "grow up" and that I have enough time left to enjoy being me and that the fears and depression and isolation never overwhelm my mind again. On the basis of past experience, I suppose that's a lot to ask—but who would have believed that I would have two kids of my own either! I hope that everyone who is trapped in anorexia nervosa or any other "lonely obsessive trap", and who realizes their misery and wants to escape, finds someone to trust and help them, as I did.'

Women suffering from bulimia nervosa may neglect their children and have difficulty forming a good relationship with them. For example, in order not to be disturbed during an eating binge, she may put her child in a separate room and close the door so that she can ignore their cries. In the longer term, women who have recovered from bulimia nervosa tend to be overly anxious about their child's weight and appearance, which may in turn affect the child's development. The problems of juggling bulimia with the needs of school-aged children are shown by Esther (in *Patient's perspective* below), who permitted us to have access to her diary after seeking help for the first time.

 Patient's perspective

'I'll do it in the morning, stomach too sore, I'm too lethargic and miserable after today's episode. Panic—another birthday party invitation. Will the kids get to go to this one or can I avoid getting out of the car to pick them up. "Mummy is always sick," they say. Sean and Angeline asked if we could go to gym on Saturday or Sunday to visit our old friends. Promised, and lied as usual, as if!!

Didn't take Sean to soccer training, couldn't bring myself to go out of the house.

It's Thursday and wow, I haven't binged since Monday, keep it up. Panic, the days are getting warmer, and soon I'll have to drop the "hiding" clothes (to avoid my fatness and shape to be seen by others).

The kids' sports carnival tomorrow, don't know what to do, I have to go, but I'm terrified. I don't want anyone to see me, and the way people look at me!! I feel so scared and vulnerable when I look like this. Three days and haven't binged or eaten anything bad, except I ate enough vegetable stir fry to feed an army.

Asked kids how they would feel if I couldn't make it to the sports carnival—very upset. I'll have to go, just grin and bear it. Took Sean to training tonight, actually got out of the car to pick him up. Angeline does gym but she meets me at the car just outside, can't wait to watch her again like I used to. So frustrated, what madness!

Sports carnival day has arrived, have to go, it's going to be so hot today and I'm wearing winter clothes. How am I going to face today. I have been eating good, not bingeing most of the week and I feel fatter than I did at the beginning of the week. Why do I always go through this transition of looking worse before I look better; but I feel better.

I actually went to the sports carnival, and lived through it, ha!! Looking around I didn't really feel like I looked different to everyone else, except more shy than usual. I have been eating a good three meals a day, except maybe too many vegetables, but at least it's only vegetables.

Day number seven. I actually thought I had this good eating down to a T—but what happened today: well I couldn't pick the kids up from school, couldn't step out of the house. I ate everything that contained fat. I made sure of that. Dad picked the kids up for me (the car was overheating) ha ha. I was too disgusted to go out, my stomach too stretched to breath properly, all I could do was lay down and panic, full of panic, my mind ached with panic, what have I done and I know Dad will be here soon and my sisters just happened to pop over—that's all I needed. I had to control the kids, which I feel I can never do properly, hold back the tears, and control the panic till they left. I have left it too long, how am I going to bring it all up now, well I tried anyway, tried being the operative word. I have become hopeless at this for some reason, even though the belts I use seem to reach half way down my throat, to the point that it bleeds and is sore for days.

I should be taking Sean to study group this afternoon but how can I drag myself out of the house—by this stage I'm in a hysterical cry, panic, frenzy; you see I'm not that successful at bringing it up. My sister's son goes to study group and she just happens to ring and ask if I would like her to pick Sean up and take him, great, he doesn't miss out. Homework, the kids, can't concentrate on anything but my disgusting, pitiful, poor excuse for a mother.

Try again tomorrow.

Who wants to wake up?

Well, it is inevitable, I had to wake up this morning, car isn't going that well so I ring my sister to take the kids to school. I would have loved to go with them today to buy them some books which are on sale this week at the school library, but instead I pack some money in their pockets and off they go, mummy's car isn't working well you see—ha!

Another excuse, I'm full of them.'

5

Investigation of eating disorders

> ## Key points
>
> - Investigation consists of a thorough physical examination and clinical history
>
> - Motivation and the advantages of maintaining the eating disorder need to be assessed
>
> - A current and past history of eating-disordered behaviour, thoughts, and beliefs are needed
>
> - Assessment includes the woman's health, family, relationships, and social history
>
> - Other medical, psychological, and psychiatric illnesses can be treated concurrently

> 'I don't want to be like this, but what I eat still rules my life so that at times every waking minute seems occupied with thoughts of food and the day passes in the measured times between when I last ate and when I'll eat again. I'm still plagued with guilt about everything I consume unless I nearly starve. I dream of the perfect day when I have no appetite, no thought, desire, or temptation for food or to eat. I often despair of ever finding a solution.'

Diagnosis and co-morbidity

The reason for making a diagnosis of an eating disorder is to enable the person to obtain treatment that is appropriate for them at the time. This can be done by obtaining a good history and by a thorough physical examination by a doctor. At times it can be difficult to know whether the symptoms belong to an eating-disorder diagnosis, are part of another medical or psychiatric illness, or are simply normal adolescent behaviour.

Many women who have an eating disorder show clinical signs of depression, and when the woman first presents asking for help, it may be unclear whether the depression led to the eating disorder or if the eating disorder led to the depression. In most cases, the two occur together and improve or disappear with nutritional rehabilitation. Examples of reasons health professionals have given to patients for not being referred for assessment of an eating disorder are given in the box below.

 Fact!

Eating-disorder sufferers can have other medical and psychiatric problems.

Examples of reasons given for not referring patients for an assessment of their eating disorder

- ◆ Weight loss is a result of major depression or viral illness

- ◆ Weight gain is a result of medication or pregnancy

- ◆ Binge eating and vomiting only followed gastric lap-banding

- ◆ Not worried about body image, only about control of eating

- ◆ No distorted body image; knows she is thin and wants to gain weight

- ◆ Has regular menstrual periods so cannot have anorexia nervosa

- ◆ Irregular menstrual periods due to polycystic ovarian syndrome

- ◆ Has diabetes; has coeliac disease; has Turner's syndrome; has food allergies

- ◆ Has depression; has Asperger's disorder; abuses drugs or alcohol

Physical examination

This examination includes careful measurements of the person's weight and height, so that the body mass index (BMI) can be calculated (see pages 22 and 36). Signs that can be observed when examining a person suffering from an eating disorder are shown in the box below.

External signs of patients with an eating disorder

- Body weight (under- or overweight)

- Clothing loose or tight (reflecting weight change or to disguise it)

- Dry skin (dehydration), sometimes yellow from carotenaemia

- Overdeveloped muscles (excessive exercise)

- Excessive hairiness (lanugo), especially on the face and forearms (underweight)

- Calluses on the back of hands and fingers (from inducing vomiting)

- Fingers and face puffy (binge eating)

- Enlarged parotid glands (vomiting)

- Peripheral oedema (multiple reasons)

- Teeth discoloured and damaged (vomiting and poor nutrition)

- Hands and feet cold and blue

The physical examination and investigation will depend upon the clinical presentation and history. The essentials are given in the box below. Additional tests that may be suggested are: cholesterol and triglycerides if the woman is obese, serum amylase if self-induced vomiting is suspected, and bone mineral density if the woman is of low body weight.

Minimal physical examination and investigations

Body height and weight	Phosphate
Serum ferritin	Blood glucose
Heart rate	Liver function tests
Calcium	Serum electrolytes
Blood pressure	Thyroid function
Magnesium	Serum creatinine
Full blood count	Electrocardiogram

Advantages of an eating disorder

Most people with eating disorders have poor self-esteem and a poor body image. For this reason, it is important for the health professional to make a psychological evaluation of the woman before starting any treatment. One purpose of asking questions is to try to establish whether the patient is prepared to alter her eating behaviour, to lose or gain weight, and if she has sufficiently high motivation and resilience to make the changes. If her motivation is low, or her perceived advantages of continuing her eating disorder outweigh the disadvantages, a great deal of time will be expended, both by the health professional and the patient, with little benefit until these issues are addressed. The advantages vary and can depend on whether the person has anorexia nervosa, bulimia nervosa, or is severely obese at the time. Possible advantages are shown in the box below.

 Fact!

There are advantages to having an eating disorder:

- To avoid having to make decisions

- To avoid the age-related challenges that are normally experienced

- To avoid sexual feelings and relationships

- To elicit care and contact with family members

- To feel loved and looked after by the family

- To keep the family together and communicating

- To avoid going out and attending social functions

- To avoid competition

- To have an excuse not to be perfect

- To make their partner feel needed

- To stop others picking on them or bullying them

- To feel part of the family by looking like them (physically)

- To feel in control (of life, feelings, weight, eating)

- To stop feeling as much, to cover sad emotions

- To feel something

- To stop feeling empty inside

- To flatten swings in mood

- To cope with forthcoming events, such as an exam

- Because it is familiar and predictable; to feel safe

- To be the best at something

- To feel a sense of achievement

- To be what their partner desires

- To get help for problems experienced

- To get help for a parent or partner

One patient said: '*When my body weight is normal I am scared of people's expectations of me, and have to resist men who make advances. But when I am fat, I am able to avoid these problems.*' Another patient used her illness to justify her behaviour towards her husband, saying: '*My husband knew that he was marrying a sick person. If I get better, he may not like me and we may separate.*'

 Patient's perspective

One of our patients ceased competitive swimming at the age of 12 and began putting on weight.

'All the girls were too competitive. I'm out of that now and can get on with everyone. When I was swimming, people picked on me if I didn't do as well as they expected me to have done. Now I can do what I like, and do the things I like well. Now I'm fat, I find that people come and talk to me. They can see I have a problem. They can see I have a weakness of character, or I wouldn't eat so much. They have problems too. Other people can't see their problems, but as my problem is obvious, they feel comfortable with me.'

Some women feel a sense of achievement in being able to reduce their weight so that they become emaciated. One of our patients, aged 20, who had anorexia nervosa and who had, in her words, done nothing with her life, wrote to us saying: '*At least I've done one thing well. I enjoy being my doctor's worst patient.*'

Suggestion: Make a list of the advantages and disadvantage of keeping your eating disorder.

Current assessment of the eating disorder

The eating and exercise Quality of Life for Eating Disorders (QOL ED, see page 229) is a quick 31-question self-report assessing:

◆ eating behaviour;

◆ disordered-eating feelings;

◆ psychological feelings;

◆ the affect of eating and exercise on daily life (relationships, work or study, social);

- the affect of eating and exercise on medical status;

- body weight;

- overeating feelings;

- exercise feelings; and

- global score.

The QOL ED can be used to discuss with the patient their current areas of distress and to clarify any misconceptions the patient may have about their understanding of their eating disorder or their medical health. Later, the QOL ED can be used to assess and discuss progress. There are many other assessment tools, such as the Eating Disorder Examination (EDE), but these do not include quality-of-life measures.

Clinical history

The clinical examination includes the current assessment. The following 20 questions have been found to be helpful for health professionals in establishing someone's motivation, as well as providing information for planning treatment. Patients can find it helpful to write down their answer to each question and read it again a week or two later and discuss their reactions with their therapist.

This history seeks information about what supports the woman has, her family and work expectations and aspirations, and those of her family and friends. It explores her beliefs, behaviours and attitudes to eating, her weight, and her life in general.

1. Do you really want to change your eating behaviour, have you tried?

 Fact!

It may take months or years before a patient is able to accept or participate actively in treatment.

Suggestion: Try to change your behaviour to prove to yourself you can.

2. What is your occupation?

Suggestions:

Try to avoid places and part-time jobs associated with food and exercise.

Try to avoid jobs that disrupt regular structured eating patterns, e.g. shift work, travel.

Occupations involving certain body image requirements may make recovery difficult.

3. What weight would you like to achieve?

 Fact!

Most women with an eating disorder will desire an unrealistic body weight.

4. What is the lightest and the heaviest weight you have ever been?

 Fact!

Some individuals can have more than one type of eating disorder in their lifetime.

5. Have you maintained your weight over a period of at least 6 months without much effort?

Suggestion: Introduce the concept of a desirable weight range as defined by a BMI rather than a single weight.

6. How do you think changing your weight will change your lifestyle?

Suggestion: Make a list of the reasons why you want to gain or to lose weight.

7. **What do you think would happen to your weight if you ate 'normally'?**

 Fact!

Most eating-disorder patients overestimate or underestimate how much they need to eat.

8. **Have you previously tried dieting to lose or to gain weight?**

Suggestion: List and write about the reasons you were not successful.

9. **Have you used any other ways, apart from dieting and exercise, to lose weight?**

Fact!

All eating-disorder patients can use extreme measures from time to time (see box below).

List of potentially dangerous weight-losing behaviours

- Self-induced vomiting
- Vomiting induced by emetics
- Misuse of laxatives
- Misuse of thyroid hormones
- Misuse of diuretics (fluid tablets)
- Excessive exercising
- Prescribed drugs, usually stimulants
- Party drugs, usually stimulants

- Other social drugs including nicotine

- Insulin misuse by diabetic women

- Food misuse by women with coeliac disease

10. If you keep to your menu plan, how quickly do you think that you will gain weight or will lose weight?

Suggestion: Expect eating and exercise plans to need regular modification during treatment.

11. Do you do regular exercise?

 Fact!

Regular enjoyable exercise is beneficial but excessive inappropriate exercise is unhealthy (see *Patient's perspective*: Belinda, Chapter 2).

12. Are you taking any medication at present?

 Fact!

Patients with eating disorders can have other medical and psychiatric problems.

Patients with eating disorders often take vitamins, herbs and 'natural' remedies.

13. Do you use any social drugs, including caffeine, alcohol, or nicotine?

14. Tell me about your family.

 Fact!

A thorough family history is necessary, including roles, appearances and dynamics.

15. Tell me about your lifestyle.

 Fact!

Most patients with eating disorders need to modify the structure of their daily living to recover.

16. How do you feel about yourself?

 Fact!

Eating disorders are associated with a low self-esteem.

17. When did you have your last menstrual period?

 Fact!

A thorough health history of the woman, including sexuality, is necessary.

Suggestion: Plot your weight, eating behaviour, and self-esteem since first menstruation.

18. Have you ever had any unpleasant experiences including bullying, physical or sexual abuse, being threatened or been in fear of your life, or being constantly criticised?

 Fact!

Physical and sexual abuse influences the severity and outcome of eating disorders.

19. Have you had any problems becoming pregnant?

 Fact!

Fertility problems occur in women with eating disorders (see Chapter 4).

20. Have any of your family been treated for any psychological or psychiatric problems?

 Fact!

Eating disorders and other psychiatric problems occur more often in families.

Different family members or relatives can have different eating disorders.

6

General management of eating disorders

> ## ➔ Key points
>
> - The aims of management are to help the person have a good quality of life that is free of eating-disordered thoughts and behaviours
>
> - The types of management range from self-help with no support to inpatient hospital treatment with maximum supervision and help from a multidisciplinary team
>
> - The dietician is an integral part of management and establishing 'normal' structured eating; this includes addressing faulty beliefs and misconceptions
>
> - A mood and food diary provides information and is an essential treatment tool
>
> - Supportive psychotherapy forms the basis for ongoing psychological treatment
>
> - A variety of other psychological therapies, including cognitive behaviour therapy, are employed depending on a person's age, stage of illness, type of disorder, and her past and present problems

'When this all started, I used to always use a knife to eat an apple, and a teaspoon to eat cereal or dessert—I suppose it took longer and therefore I felt as if I was eating more. I always left a bit of potato/rice/noodles on my plate, no matter how much was served—as a test of willpower. The whole exercise of putting on weight, to me, is a breakdown of my iron willpower, because I know only too well that I enjoy eating. That is what still revolts me—the amount of food actually to be consumed in order to put on the weight. I've always maintained that I would so much prefer to have the weight "sewn" on instead of having to "eat" it on.'

Aims of treatment

The aims of the treatment for someone with an eating disorder are:

1. To persuade her to achieve and accept a weight that lies in the normal range (BMI 19–24.9), or a higher realistic weight if she is obese.

2. To help her to learn or relearn 'normal eating' patterns.

3. To help her gain insight into her eating behaviour and why the behaviour is persisting.

4. To educate her about nutrition and normal eating, and to dispel misconceptions about food and eating.

5. To persuade her to stop using behaviours that are potentially dangerous or unhelpful.

6. To help her learn to cope with the problems in her life that may be aggravating the eating behaviour or preventing her recovery.

7. To help her alter or modify her lifestyle, as appropriate, to aid recovery.

For a person to change from having an eating disorder to learning or returning to 'normal' eating depends on the person making several decisions:

1. She must accept that she has an eating disorder.

2. She must believe that, if the disordered eating continues, it may cause a serious problem to her lifestyle and/or to her health.

3. She must want to improve her quality of life with regard to eating and exercise.

4. She must accept the help given, but understand that the change will only occur if she is prepared to achieve the change herself.

Suggestion: Complete the QOL ED before commencing treatment and every 3 months (see Appendix C).

This means she has to decide that the benefits or rewards of changing her disordered-eating behaviour exceed the cost of continuing with it, at a physical, psychological, and social level. Having made these decisions, she has to show a readiness to change her present eating habits.

Choosing the type of management

Once the woman has accepted that she has an eating disorder and has decided to seek help, the next step is to find out about the different types of treatment, and which are available and accessible. Information is available for patients and their families from friends and relatives, books, and the Internet. Before making a decision, the options should be discussed with the woman's family doctor following a physical and psychological assessment. An assessment should always be sought, even if self-help methods (see Table 6.1) are initially preferred. *Physical and psychological assessments can determine the most appropriate treatment.*

Using a self-help manual under the guidance of a therapist or family doctor overcomes many of the criticisms of the self-help method. Guided self-help improves compliance with treatment, provides support for dealing with unwanted emotions, and ensures continuing assessment and follow-up. The great advantage is that this method can be used by people with limited access to treatment, as support can be provided by email. The level of 'drop out' from self-help treatment is greater if the participant has unrealistic expectations and goals.

Once the information is obtained and the patient is open to receiving professional treatment, several options are available. The helpers may be the person's family doctor, a psychiatrist, a dietician, an eating-disorder specialist, or a multidisciplinary team (which generally includes a dietician, a psychologist, and a medical specialist). The option that is most appropriate will differ from person to person. If the woman's health is so bad that admission to hospital is required, the most successful results occur if she is admitted to a specialized eating-disorders unit. The various options available are given in Table 6.2.

Beliefs and misconceptions

The treatment of eating disorders is more complicated than weight change and weight stabilization. The acquisition of unhelpful beliefs and thinking are part of developing and maintaining an eating disorder. The box below contains some statements patients report as 'normal' eating. Treatment includes challenging and modifying these inappropriate thoughts and practices. Normal eating is described in Chapter 10.

Table 6.1 Advantages and disadvantages of different types of self-help management

Method	Advantages	Disadvantages
Self-help manuals	• Useful for patients who are well-motivated and not emaciated, grossly obese, or very unwell in the first instance • It is a fast way of getting information and collecting knowledge about healthy eating behaviour • Can be used by people living in areas where no eating-disorder treatment is available	• It is very difficult to deal with established eating problems alone • Patients lose their ability to assess their weight properly • Patients get frustrated as improvement does not occur as fast as they expect or wish it to • Patients have to deal with the feelings that arise in response to changes in behaviour by themselves • It is easy to be distracted and lose motivation and hope
Self-help support groups	• Groups that are well organized provide help to many women • Leaders of the group who are partially or fully recovered from an eating disorder can provide hope for change • People can find being part of a group less intimidating than seeing a therapist • The positive milieu of the group can support the recovery process • People feel that they can overcome the eating disorder by themselves • Good support groups provide 'emergency' numbers in case patients experience crises	• Members can teach each other bad habits • People can compete to be the best or worst in the group • The group might reinforce the preoccupation with weight, food, and exercise because of conversations held in the group • Sometimes no routine assessment procedures exist to determine whether a person needs to seek the help of a medical or other specialist, or would benefit from a different treatment • Some people do not like the idea of group participation • Some groups condone excessive disordered exercise as a form of recovery

(continued)

Table 6.1 Advantages and disadvantages of different types of self-help management *(continued)*

Method	Advantages	Disadvantages
Internet support	• Is an easy accessible medium • People in isolated areas (e.g. Australia or Canada), with no easy access to doctors/specialists, can be reached and can get advice from experts • The anonymity of patients is guaranteed • Information can prevent people spending money on useless 'magical cures' • Chat lines are useful for finding out about good care, e.g. bariatric surgeons providing multidisciplinary care	• Destructive content can exist on sites that are not supervised by professionals • A few sites actively promote anorexia nervosa, bulimia nervosa, and obesity • Bad habits and 'magical cures' (e.g. techniques for vomiting) can be spread more easily through the Internet • Patients may take information out of context

Table 6.2 Advantages and disadvantages of the different treatment options and who is most suitable for each treatment

Treatment	Who is suitable	Advantages	Disadvantages
Outpatient treatment	• Obese patients, most bulimia nervosa patients, and some anorexia nervosa patients	• Does not interfere with studies or work • Patients are with their families and friends • Patients are making changes as part of their normal daily living • Patients can feel in control of their treatment	• The challenges of everyday situations can be difficult to manage • In problem situations or crises, patients are often overwhelmed

(continued)

Table 6.2 Advantages and disadvantages of the different treatment options and who is most suitable for each treatment *(continued)*

Treatment	Who is suitable	Advantages	Disadvantages
Partial hospitalization or day-patient treatment	◆ Patients following treatment in hospital ◆ Patients needing more support and treatment than is provided as an outpatient ◆ Outpatients with recent severe weight loss or weight gain ◆ Relapsing patients	◆ Good for assisting with the transition from inpatient to outpatient treatment ◆ Offers containment and supervision of behaviours for some meals, but allows the patient to take responsibility for others ◆ Themes that were raised and addressed during outpatient or inpatient individual and/or group therapy can be continued ◆ Provides group support	◆ Few research studies about the effectiveness of day-patient treatment exist ◆ No proven regimen for day-patient treatment ◆ A relatively high number of patients with anorexia nervosa lose weight during day-patient treatment ◆ Not successful for patients with unrealistic expectations of weight loss ◆ Time away, from work, and study
Inpatient treatment	◆ Patients who experience frequent relapses ◆ Patients who have a medical condition or are medically unwell ◆ Patients who have co-morbid psychiatric conditions	◆ Medical conditions are better controlled and treated ◆ A structured environment with supervision supports healthy eating behaviour ◆ Support and help exist on a 24-hour basis	◆ Patients have to make the transition from the structure and support of the hospital to their home and daily lives ◆ Some patients have difficulties being separated from their family or partner, especially when they live far away from the hospital

(continued)

Table 6.2 Advantages and disadvantages of the different treatment options and who is most suitable for each treatment (*continued*)

Treatment	Who is suitable	Advantages	Disadvantages
Inpatient treatment (*continued*)	◆ Patients who live in areas where treatment is not available ◆ Patient or family preference ◆ Patients whose living environment is reinforcing the disorder	◆ Can provide temporary relief from a stressful psychosocial environment (e.g. family, work) ◆ Patients have others to talk to and share their thoughts and feelings with ◆ Provides treatment for a range of other problems	◆ Patients who experience more support inside than outside hospital may continue their unhelpful behaviours

How women with an eating disorder describe 'normal' eating

◆ 'When in company, eating slowly and finishing last.'

◆ 'Seeing how long I can stretch out the meal.'

◆ 'When alone, eating quickly so that I get rid of it and don't enjoy it.'

◆ 'Saying no to food.'

◆ 'Filling up on fluids before meals.'

◆ 'Cutting up and dissecting my food to show I am in control.'

◆ 'Sticking to rigid eating times—too bad if you miss it.'

◆ 'Only eating healthy foods.'

◆ 'Only eating fat-free foods.'

◆ 'Disguising the flavour of tasty foods so that they taste nasty.'

- 'Going on an eating binge.'

- 'Making food the focus of my day.'

- 'Always having food available.'

Nutritional management

The dietician is an integral part of management. Because patients with eating disorders usually have unhelpful ideas about the nature of the foods they eat, or do not eat, and because one of the aims of treatment is to restore normal eating behaviour, a dietician is an important member of the team. The role of the dietician is described in the box below.

What does a dietician do?

- Takes an accurate history of the patients eating and fluid intake behaviour

- Helps to set up a healthy and well-balanced meal plan

- Explains the nutritional content of food and provides information about basic nutritional matters

- Educates about normal eating and dispels myths about food and eating

- Supports the patient to develop a normal attitude to food and to establish an appropriate eating behaviour

- Helps to stop behaviours that are potentially dangerous

- Helps to structure eating behaviour and to set up strategies for restoring weight to, or maintaining, an appropriate weight

- Encourages the patient to start a food diary for 7 days describing foods that have been eaten, fluids drunk, and where and when

- Helps gain insight into the eating behaviour and why the behaviour is persisting

- Helps with advice on how to maintain weight within a healthy weight range

- Helps introduce previously 'banned' foods into the menu plan

 Fact!

Patients with eating disorders have disordered drinking patterns.

Daily diaries and planning

One important adjunct to treatment is the use of diaries, with different records kept for different purposes. The first diary is usually a daily record of everything the woman is eating and drinking, the exercise she is taking, and how she is feeling at the time (see Table 6.3). This helps the dietician to set realistic short-term goals and devise a suitable menu plan in conjunction with the woman. Once the itemized food record is no longer needed, the eating behaviour should be monitored in more general terms to ensure that the woman's preoccupation with thoughts of food and energy are not reinforced unnecessarily.

In the treatment of eating disorders, the daily diary allows the woman to:

- gain insight into the associations between her feelings, moods, and eating behaviour;

- observe and monitor changes in her eating and associated behaviours;

- plan and make changes to her lifestyle that will promote recovery.

The diary monitors and provides information about:

- the woman's perception of her over- or undereating;

- her over- and underdrinking;

- her eating pattern throughout the day (structured or chaotic);

- her feelings around eating episodes;

Table 6.3 Example of a mood, food, and exercise diary

Day of week:					
Date:					
Time and place	Type of eating or exercise*	Food eaten or exercise done	Behaviour	Thoughts and feelings at the time	Thoughts and feelings later

* e.g. snack, binge, and indicate any weight loss method.

- her binge eating or overeating episodes (time of day, time of month);

- her patterns of weight-losing behaviour;

- her exercise patterns;

- her lifestyle (regular, structured, or spontaneous);

- her moods and mood changes (including precipitants);

- her alcohol and drug use;

- her ability to fulfil a task;

- her motivation to change.

The diary can also be used in the treatment of other associated problems, such as reducing obsessional behaviours, working through unhelpful thought patterns, and looking at events that may be maintaining disordered behaviour. Often, when a patient feels that she is not improving in spite of treatment, checking back in the diary and talking about it shows that her feelings can mislead her and that in fact she is improving.

Psychological treatment

Supportive psychotherapy forms the basis for treatment. Other psychological treatments are available in a variety of methods. One of these, cognitive behavioural therapy, has given superior results, particularly for bulimia nervosa. Seldom is only one type of psychological treatment employed by therapists, and most patients will experience a more eclectic management of their eating disorder and related problems. This individualized, flexible approach includes cognitive behavioural therapy, family therapy, interpersonal therapy, behaviour therapy, mindfulness, acceptance and commitment therapy, dialectical behaviour therapy, and schema therapy. With this approach to treating eating disorders, superior results are achieved, possibly because the therapy can be fitted to the individual patient, the stage in their illness, their age, and their living environment. Dialectical behaviour therapy and schema approaches are used for patients with personality problems and borderline personality disorder.

Table 6.4 gives an overview of some of the most common psychological therapy techniques that are used in the treatment of eating disorders. In fact, many of these therapies are based on cognitive behaviour therapy and contain techniques from some of the older therapies such as relaxation, motivation, and hypnosis.

Table 6.4. Psychological therapy techniques used in the treatment of eating disorders

Therapy	Techniques used
Supportive psychotherapy	◆ Provides reassurance, advice and guidance, and encourages the patient to take responsibility for change
	◆ Encourages expression of feelings and emotional material
	◆ Helps the patients to understand what is happening
	◆ Examines the patient's individual problems and needs
	◆ Aims to teach coping strategies for different, mainly stressful, situations without relapsing into old behaviours
	◆ Provides intervention when crises occur
	◆ Is the main therapy during and after other interventions
	◆ Is mostly used in individual therapy
Cognitive behavioural therapy	◆ Focuses on bringing about changes in negative thought patterns
	◆ Identifies the beliefs of the person that influence how they experience and deal with daily living
	◆ Helps the person to understand how these beliefs affect their reactions
	◆ Provides an understanding of how these beliefs help to maintain the disordered eating
	◆ Challenges these beliefs by doing behavioural experiments
	◆ Is used in individual and group therapy

(continued)

Table 6.4. Psychological therapy techniques used in the treatment of eating disorders *(continued)*

Therapy	Techniques used
Family therapy	• Useful for treating eating disorders in young people aged 16 years or below
	• Assessment of the family and partial involvement in therapy should be considered in older patients, particularly if they are still living at home
	• Aims to: (i) help the therapist and family understand the family dynamics and the reasons for the eating disorder; (ii) help the family members develop an understanding for the behaviour of the eating-disordered member of the family; and (iii) help the family learn how to provide support for the sufferer in the recovery process
Interpersonal psychotherapy	• Therapy sessions focus on one of four interpersonal problem areas (grief, role conflict, interpersonal conflict, and social deficit)
	• Concentrates on depression, which occurs as a result of a problem in one or more of the above-mentioned interpersonal conflict areas
	• Is one of the few empirically validated types of psychotherapy that addresses the problem, provides insight, and promotes action and problem-solving
	• Is used in short-term individual therapy (12–15 sessions)
Dialectical behavioural therapy	• Sets boundaries for behaviour
	• Promotes a balance between acceptance and change through regular monitoring of behaviours and emotional and cognitive states
	• Promotes practise in mindfulness and improving the skills of managing emotions
	• Promotes improvements in interpersonal relationships and toleration of distress
	• Is used in individual and group therapy for personality disorder

(continued)

Table 6.4. Psychological therapy techniques used in the treatment of eating disorders (*continued*)

Therapy	Techniques used
Mindfulness-based cognitive therapy	◆ Focuses on learning coping strategies to be able to stay in the present moment/situation when exposed to unpleasant emotions
	◆ Teaches how to be mindful of thoughts, thinking patterns, and behaviour, and to use this mindfulness to get through a certain situation or emotion
	◆ Helps to learn relaxation and mindful eating
	◆ Is used in individual and group therapy
Acceptance and commitment therapy	◆ Assumes many psychological problems and feelings resulting from fear
	◆ Helps people accept their reactions and feel them, and not to try and avoid or change them, including old and new experiences and trauma
	◆ Promotes recognizing and clarifying personal values and taking action on these, creating a meaningful life
Schema therapy	◆ Assumes that maladaptive coping styles (schemas) relate to childhood experiences
	◆ Helps to provide insight into feelings and to learn new ways of coping
	◆ Helps find constructive ways of meeting emotional needs
	◆ Helps in the adjustment and acceptance of early life experiences

7

Anorexia nervosa and anorexia nervosa-like disorders

→ Key points

- The incidence of anorexia nervosa is not increasing; rather there is a increasing recognition of anorexia in the community

- The onset of anorexia nervosa usually occurs in adolescent women after first menstruation

- The triggers for onset of the illness may not be the same as those that perpetuate the behaviour and those that prevent recovery

- The physical and psychological symptoms of anorexia nervosa are those of starvation and sometimes extreme weight-losing behaviour

- The anorexia nervosa sufferer is disabled by her preoccupation with disordered thoughts about eating, food, weight, and weight loss

- Patients with anorexia nervosa have disordered drinking behaviour and fluid intake

- The occurrence of the menstrual cycle depends on adequate energy stores—in the form of fat—in the body; this also applies to first menstruation

- The incidence of anorexia nervosa is less than 1%, and that of anorexia nervosa-like disorders may be as high as 3–4%

'I just wish that anorexia would get the blazes out of my life! Everything I do, have done or didn't do centres around my fear of food. For those of you not familiar with the demonic workings of anorexia, fear of food and getting fat are its basic elements.'

Description

The classical sufferer is female and has completed puberty. Onset occurs during adolescence following a weight loss, although the eating disorder may not become apparent for several years. The initial weight loss may be intentional and in response to post-pubertal weight gain, or it may occur for other reasons such as illness or a change in exercise routine. Following significant weight loss, women, particularly if they have a genetic sensitivity, can become preoccupied with thoughts that make them unable to accept the feelings they experience while gaining their body weight back to a 'normal' healthy range. The definition and diagnostic criteria for anorexia nervosa were discussed in Chapter 2.

Demographics

'Anorexia now seems to be becoming increasingly common, and receiving a lot of publicity. I don't know whether the publicity is all for the good—I have the feeling it may be becoming almost "fashionable" among young girls, without their realising its long-term consequences. If I could but turn the clock back about 12 years—wishful thinking!'

In spite of media hype, anorexia nervosa is not occurring in epidemic proportions and the numbers remain fairly constant (see box below). What has changed over the last 30 years is the increasing recognition of anorexia nervosa among members of the community and greater access to treatment. We have also become increasingly aware there are many young women in the community who have a short period of anorexia nervosa behaviour and thinking, and who 'recover' without treatment or with minimal intervention by their family, school teachers, or family doctor. A few children under the age of 13 and men also develop anorexia nervosa.

Demographics of anorexia nervosa

- Lifetime prevalence of 0.3–1.0%

- New cases each year are around 8 per 100,000 of the population

- Predominately occurs in post-pubertal women

- Peak incidence is 14–18 years

- Onset usually occurs during adolescence

- Estimated to have a 50–80% genetic component

- Occurs across all socioeconomic groups

- Occurs among different cultures, although the presentations may vary

- Most cases are not assessed or treated by mental health professionals

- Other co-morbid medical and psychiatric illnesses can exist

- Time for recovery is very variable, usually within 5 years

- Most people recover and have a good quality of life

The estimated prevalence for anorexia nervosa and anorexia nervosa-like disorders is 3–4%.

Onset

Weight loss at the onset of anorexia nervosa may not be intentional and can follow a decision by the woman to eat 'healthily' and improve her fitness, or may follow a series of events that are stressful in themselves, such as a break-up with a boyfriend, an unwanted pregnancy, a major examination, or a period of further deterioration in already stressful circumstances such as parents separating.

 Fact!

Initial weight loss may not be due to body image concerns.

The onset of anorexia nervosa seldom occurs for the first time after the age of 40 unless in the context of medical- or psychiatric-initiated weight loss. Even among women who appear to have their onset in their later 20s and 30s, their history is likely to include concerns about weight or eating, such as maintaining a low weight with restrictive eating patterns, disordered eating behaviour, the presence of another eating disorder including obesity, excessive exercise, or another medical or psychiatric illness.

Maintaining anorexia nervosa

Young women can have a transitory experience with anorexia nervosa behaviour and thinking, yet not all go on to have an eating disorder requiring treatment by mental health professionals. Why some people continue with their eating-disorder behaviour and why a few develop a chronic condition is not clear. Genetic factors play a part, as well as ongoing problems associated with unpleasant, depressive, or anxious feelings.

Family stress may be important. Adolescence is a time of struggle for independence from parents and mixed messages can be given, for example, 'You must be independent but we need you at home.' If one or both parents are overcontrolling, the young woman can be confused, wanting to be independent but feeling unable to escape the enmeshment of the family. In other instances, the young woman may find she is lacking support and has no role models or carers. This can happen when one parent leaves or becomes ill, and the young woman becomes the confidant and support person for her parent or feels rejected by a parent for a new partner.

Restricting food can help a woman feel in control of her feelings and her life, and can decrease the intensity of her uncomfortable and confusing feelings. As body weight decreases, the illness becomes self-perpetuating for both physiological and psychological reasons.

Preoccupation with food and fear of gaining weight

Preoccupation with thoughts of food and weight leads anorexia nervosa patients to use a range of behaviours to achieve their desire (see *Patient's perspective*: Cassandra).

Patient's perspective

The fear of losing control, confusion, and preoccupation with control over weight and food are captured by Cassandra in her diary when her BMI was 15:

'My arms are so flabby, my stomach huge, and I am really getting worried because lunch is coming up. I really wanted Mum to help me think I can eat it, but she's gone now and I feel so sick I cannot face food. I know I should have it, but something deep inside me tells me not to—I really want to listen to it because I know it will help me feel better later—and help my problems (i.e. FATNESS!). I'm worried Mum is going to get me lunch or ask me what I want and I don't know whether I'm hungry or not yet. I need someone to help me decide and understand. I feel very bad because I didn't go for a walk this morning and the fact that I have time to go now and haven't yet makes it even worse. I'm very tired and don't think I will go—but I know I'll be punished with FATNESS for that. I don't know why I don't avoid that consequence and go—but I really don't think I can.'

'I have been having very bad thoughts again and have wanted to die. Last night I took out a lot of laxatives and other fat stopping pills but Mum came into my room before I took them. They are in my box now—and I am worried I might take too many one day. I put the scales back in my room because I have to monitor my weight closely at the moment as I have lost a little weight yet I know I am fatter, which is confusing me, and so I think I should keep an eye on the scales to see what is happening to me.'

'Dieters and exercisers'

This group of patients with anorexia nervosa, comprising young women whose weight is usually in the normal range before their eating disorder, generally begin losing weight by the simple method of eating less, eating 'healthily', and by avoiding situations in which they have to eat. In order to avoid eating, they make excuses such as '*I don't feel hungry at the moment so I'll eat some later.*' Other excuses offered include, '*I have eaten already,*' '*I've decided to become vegetarian,*' '*I have an allergy to ...*' and '*I feel sick.*' The young women tend to avoid social occasions where food is eaten. They may be competitive and are often obsessive about their studies, and they withdraw from contact with their friends. In addition to strict dieting, they may use exercise as a method of losing weight. This may involve going for a run or spending long hours at the gym. Exercise may become excessive and may become a disorder in itself (see page 31 and *Patient's perspective*: Jenny).

Patient's perspective

Jenny was 15 when she went on holiday on her own. At the holiday resort, she entered a beauty contest and came second. That night she got drunk for the first time and had her first experience of sexual intercourse. She felt guilty about being drunk and about having sex. At school, she was a good student, she worked hard, and she excelled at sports, being in the school swimming, hockey, and basketball teams. On her return from holiday, she believed that she would have won the beauty contest if she had been slimmer and if her thighs and bottom had been smaller. She decided to go on a diet to lose weight, and this resulted in arguments with her mother, who thought that Jennifer was already slim. Jenny compromised by offering to do the cooking (in reality it was to help her have control over the energy content). During meals, she moved the food about the plate so that she appeared to be eating. She avoided fatty foods, telling her family that they made her feel sick. She spent long hours alone in her room studying and in the evenings attended dancing classes. In her room, she exercised strenuously, for 15–20 minutes every 2 hours, and played music to hide the noise of her exercising from her parents. She told them that the music helped her concentrate upon her studies. She became obsessional about her weight, weighing herself before and after meals, before and after bouts of exercise, and before and after going to the toilet.

At about this time, she was chosen to represent her state in a dancing championship and increased her daily exercise. Her weight dropped from a BMI of 22 to a BMI of 18.7. She wore loose clothes to disguise her low weight from her family. As the time of the championships approached, Jenny increased the amount of exercise she did daily, and, because she still felt she was too fat, restricted her food intake still further. Two weeks before the championships, she collapsed and was admitted to hospital. Her BMI was 13.3. In hospital, she became agitated. With refeeding, she gained weight and with her parents' agreement she discharged herself from hospital. At home, she continued to exercise excessively and again collapsed.

She was readmitted to hospital and remained in hospital until her weight had increased to a BMI of 19.3.

Since discharge, she has maintained her weight at around a BMI of 18.7. Exercise has become an obsession, so much so that she jogs in the street if her doctor is running late with his appointments. However, in spite of a strenuous exercise programme, she eats sufficient food to maintain her body weight.

Potentially dangerous methods of weight control and binge eating

'Vomiters and purgers'

This second group of patients with anorexia nervosa, who may have been overweight before the start of the illness and whose weight tends to fluctuate during the illness, use potentially dangerous methods to lose weight. In public, or among the family, they may appear to eat normal amounts of food. However, having eaten, they make excuses to leave the group and induce vomiting, and may combine this with the excessive use of laxatives. Because of their eating habits, phases of severe weight reduction causing emaciation can be interspersed with periods of weight gain. They tend to be more social and less obsessional than the 'dieters and exercisers'. In some cases, the woman may have been a binge eater for several months or even years before a decision to lose weight relentlessly precipitates her into anorexia nervosa.

 Patient's perspective

Barbara thinks that she began 'binge eating' when she was 10. The binge usually consisted of eating a packet or two of biscuits, several ice creams, and whatever she could find in the house when she came home from school. By the age of 13, Barbara had begun to menstruate and her BMI was 28. In the following year, she became interested in boys, became aware that she was fat, and stopped eating sweets and cakes. She knew she was overweight, but she was popular, had an active social life, and achieved high grades at school. Over the next 5 years, her weight decreased slowly so that by the age of 18 her BMI was 25.5. At this time, problems in her parents' marriage were becoming apparent. At the end of the second year at university, she decided that she must lose weight for the coming summer and began dieting. She also avoided eating while studying. As a result, her BMI fell to 23 over a period of 4 months. She restricted her diet further, began counting calories, and started running and taking laxatives daily because of constipation. Her parents had now separated, and after trying to live with her father she moved into her mother's house. By winter, she had a BMI of 14.6 and her periods had ceased. She abused laxatives and on days of 'overeating' she would vomit afterwards. She was admitted to hospital for refeeding. When her BMI was 18.6, she was discharged 'cured of anorexia nervosa'.

Her preoccupation with being extremely thin had ceased, but she still had an eating disorder. This became apparent later that year when she went away with a group of students. She wrote to the clinic:

'I spent the first 3 weeks of the holiday trekking in the Himalayas, which are astonishingly beautiful. I was enjoying the fantastic scenery, the fresh air, and the exercise, and seemed to escape my problems up here high in the mountains. But on the last days of the trek, I got extremely sick with acute dysentery, fever—the works—doubled up by unbelievable cramps. I had to stay in bed for several weeks feeling pretty rotten. So what did I do? I ate, believe it or not! Few but ex(?) anorexics could eat with such gusto, in spite of abdominal pains, but somehow I managed and I have continued to eat since I came home. I am now even fatter than before—my BMI is 25.7 and I still have diarrhoea and cramps at times. But these will go; the tests are negative. What I'm rather distressed about is my weight (what else!) as I feel it is slowly destroying my ability to cope with everyday life. Just as my eating behaviour is out of control, my life seems to be getting the same way. My social life is eventful and fun, on the whole, and I'm not withdrawn, but I have that frantic sense of imminent doom and I'm incredibly fearful of putting on more weight. I've tried many ways to overcome whatever it is that makes me eat but I can't break the pattern for more than 2 or 3 days. I've thought of the alternatives—getting fatter, vomiting, starving—even suicide . . . but actually I'd give my right arm to have the whole lot sorted out. I'm enjoying Uni and the course, which is full of interest (when I'm not occupying my mind with stagnant thoughts of weight and food). I'd rather anything than spending half my time on food. And it was this feeling that made me diet, and become anorexic, 2 years ago.'

Anorexia nervosa in males

Anorexia nervosa occurs in males less frequently than in females (see box below). It begins in the same way, and its clinical characteristics and its course are identical to those in females. Most males with anorexia nervosa spend hours each day jogging, bodybuilding, and doing press-ups and other exercises. They are as obsessed about food and body weight as women and may become personal trainers or work in the food industry. Why males should pursue thinness so relentlessly is obscure, as adolescent men seek to be muscular rather than thin. Unlike women, men do not experience a rapid unwanted increase in body weight in early adolescence (rather, they lose body fat) or the accompanying loss of self-esteem.

Features of male patients with anorexia nervosa compared with female patients

- Less common (1 in 15 patients are male)
- More likely to be older at onset
- More likely to be heavier at onset
- More likely to induce vomiting (greater than 50%)
- More likely to binge eat before (and during)
- Much more likely to exercise excessively

It has been suggested that rates of anorexia nervosa may be higher among homosexual men but this has not been confirmed and has not been reported in previous studies of men with eating disorders. Males suffering from anorexia nervosa are likely to have additional problems including obsessive-compulsive disorder, alcohol and substance abuse, and personality disorder.

 Patient's perspective

John, aged 28, who had a 9-year history of anorexia nervosa, explained why he binge ate in a letter. After the onset of his disorder, he remained at a very low weight (BMI around 14.5) and vomited prodigiously, resulting in noticeable loss of dental enamel. Vomiting provided him with relief from anxious and depressive feelings. He was preoccupied with his binges, which were small, rather than with his vomiting.

'The result is that my tension and depression build to the point of desperation when I feel I am near insanity and even contemplate suicide. It never gets any further than this as (and I am sad to admit this, but it seems true) I end up having a binge (and I have to admit I vomit after the binge). Somehow, I end up feeling more relaxed. However, I then promise myself to make a more determined effort to beat the bingeing and the cycle starts again. This tension "build-up" cycle not only applies to my bingeing. It also applies to other projects, plans, and aspects of my life. I seem to set a goal that may be just that little bit too high for me. I don't accept myself and my own limitations. I seem to set myself up for failure. I either have to find another method of relaxation or, at least for the time being, accept my human weaknesses and, by this, I mean accept an at least limited amount of bingeing.'

Diet, and eating and drinking behaviour

As mentioned earlier, patients with anorexia nervosa are preoccupied with food. They collect and read books and magazine articles relating to food, dieting, and body weight. Often they take over the food preparation, cooking and serving food for the family. This allows the anorexic woman to control her food intake. She may also offer to do the cleaning up, which limits her time at the table, utilizes energy, and hides from her family the fact that she is not eating. In this way, her preoccupation with food continues while she is praised by her family for her helpful behaviour.

Women with anorexia nervosa read more about nutrition and food than the general public, although many of their perceptions about food are distorted and inaccurate, as much of their knowledge is used for restricting food intake, rather than for nutrition and health. Some of the false perceptions relate to the woman herself; for example, she may believe that her nutritional needs are different to other peoples or that she does not need as much food as other people.

Anorexia nervosa sufferers avoid eating all food types in their diet and avoid eating fat more than other foods. In a recent study carried out in Sydney, Australia, of 17 patients who had been ill with anorexia nervosa for less than 15 months, the diet eaten by the women at the peak of their illness was compared with that of 'normal' women of similar age. It was found to contain the following:

- one-sixth of the energy;

- one-sixth of the carbohydrates;

- one-third of the protein; and

- one-tenth of the fat.

As a group, these women showed wide variations in their nutrient intakes that reflected the beliefs they held about food at the time. The women who wanted to 'eat healthily' had even less fat in their diet. They read and remembered the information contained on food labels and a few travelled long distances to obtain food brands containing the lowest fat content.

 Fact!

Anorexia nervosa patients have disordered fluid intake behaviour.

In another study in Sydney, it was found that eating-disorder sufferers also had disordered drinking, either drinking too little to 'feel empty' and 'in control', or drinking too much to 'feel full' and prevent eating. Seldom was the intake of fluid 'normal'. More anorexia nervosa patients, particularly if they are young, have very low fluid intakes, while older patients and 'vomiters and purgers' are more likely to have excessive intakes of fluids, as drinking fluids makes it easier to vomit.

Women drinking excess amounts of fluid may dilute their blood and have low plasma sodium levels.

Biochemical changes associated with anorexia nervosa

Most of the psychological and physical changes are dependent on the biochemical changes that follow starvation, severe dieting, and dangerous methods of weight control. The main biochemical disturbances are dehydration and changes in the levels of some blood electrolytes.

The sequence of these changes is shown in Figure 7.1, which shows that, if an anorexia nervosa sufferer starves herself, induces vomiting, abuses purgatives and diuretics, or indulges in excessive exercise, she may develop a number of physical disturbances, the most serious being heart or kidney failure and death. In most cases, the changes are less life-threatening but are nevertheless disturbing to the sufferer and to her family and relatives.

Starvation or severe dieting, vomiting, laxative abuse, and excessive exercise may lead to dehydration (and low blood potassium). These are the underlying reasons for the psychological and physical symptoms that we will discuss later.

Self-induced vomiting and dehydration may cause a metabolic alkalosis, in which the woman's blood becomes alkaline due to loss of bicarbonate and a decrease in potassium and chloride. Metabolic alkalosis may impair the woman's neuromuscular function, so that she becomes easily fatigued, has muscle weakness, and may develop tingling in her hands and feet and involuntary hand clenching, which can be disturbing. More seriously, the metabolic changes may lead to an irregular heart beat and occasionally to heart failure.

A few women who abuse laxatives develop a metabolic acidosis, because of loss of bicarbonate-rich fluid in their loose stools. This may lead to hyperventilation (overbreathing) and high levels of chlorine in the blood, which very occasionally causes heart failure.

111

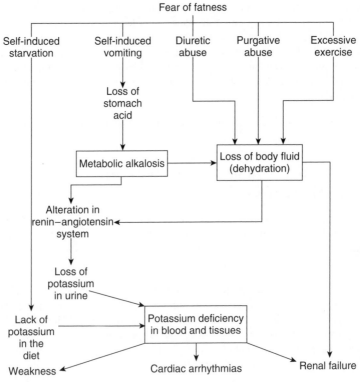

Figure 7.1 Electrolyte problems in anorexia nervosa

In spite of the severity of the weight loss or the maintenance of a very low body weight, and in spite of the use of potentially dangerous methods of weight control, it is surprising how few sufferers develop potassium deficiency (see *Patient's perspective*: Sandra). In part, this is because the body has physiological compensatory mechanisms.

 Patient's perspective

Sandra was a tall, quiet girl who was considerate, competent, and well-liked at school. When she was 14, her BMI was 23.7. She felt that she was too fat and she decided to lose weight.

Her elder sister had been told by a modelling school that one way was to induce vomiting by putting a finger down her throat. Sandra decided to do this but did not continue as little weight loss occurred. She was swimming competitively and by the age of 17, she felt fit and confident and had lost some weight (BMI 21.3).

Her 18th year was one of tragedy. Her mother was killed in a car accident, leaving two younger children. Her older sister became a drug addict and Sandra injured herself so she had to give up swimming. She deferred taking her final school exams, and took over the responsibilities of housekeeper, looking after her younger sisters. During this period, her feelings of confidence and competency disappeared. She wrote in her diary:

'I know what I should be doing. I should be going out. But meeting people is a major effort and hassle for me as I feel so uncomfortable and inept in company, especially in arranging to go to new places and meeting new people, that I end up settling for my own company. Food and eating has become such an integral part of everything.'

When she was 19, she returned to complete her final exams at the local college, where comments about her 'emaciation' induced her to eat more. Increasing her food intake was associated with episodes of binge eating, which alarmed her. She began to induce vomiting (remembering her sister's advice) by putting her fingers down her throat. Soon she was inducing vomiting up to 10 times a day. Her father found out what she was doing and insisted that she visit a doctor, who arranged for her to be admitted to hospital to help her gain weight (her BMI was 13.8) and to stop her vomiting. In hospital, she was cooperative and liked by the staff. A psychiatric consultation showed no major psychiatric illness. She was able to continue studying while in hospital and after discharge sat for and passed her exams. Her BMI was now 16.3. She persisted in dieting and in self-induced vomiting and became weak. This induced her to seek readmission to hospital. The vomiting led to a low level of potassium in her blood and tissues. She was treated with potassium supplement and an intravenous infusion.

Over the next 3 years during a university course, she had six readmissions to hospital for the effects of self-induced vomiting, low body potassium, and dehydration. These in turn caused heart-beat problems (cardiac arrhythmias) and a degree of renal failure. The admissions followed periods of increased vomiting, which Sandra related to stress from family problems. She battled against treatment saying that her illness was 'all her fault' and she resolved each day to stop vomiting. But each day she broke her resolution when she panicked about becoming fat and when she ate food. Sandra's illness became the scapegoat for the family's problems, which were considerable.

Her father remarried, and on obtaining her degree Sandra left home. Over the next 3 years, her weight increased slowly and she now has a BMI of 19. She no longer induces vomiting. When last contacted, she said, 'I look back in horror and wonder if it was some terrible nightmare.'

Hormonal changes in anorexia nervosa

Laboratory studies show that the blood levels of most hormones are lowered in anorexia nervosa, with the exception of cortisone, which is raised. One important change is that the function of the thyroid gland is reduced (hypothyroidism). This in turn leads to the slow heart rate and dry skin reported by some sufferers. The changes are due to low body weight and are not the cause of anorexia nervosa. They may be seen as the body's way of conserving energy, and hence of survival in the face of starvation.

 Fact!

When weight increases and is maintained in the normal range, all hormone levels return to normal.

Psychological disturbances in anorexia nervosa

During severe famines, as people become emaciated and biochemical changes occur, it is common to find that their personality changes and they tend to become apathetic, depressed, irritable, irrational, or emotionally labile, with violent swings in mood (see box below). These symptoms vary from day to day and week to week. Many victims of famine become obsessional, developing a preoccupation about food, or developing abnormal taste preferences. Similar psychological disturbances occur in patients with anorexia nervosa and disappear when the woman is refed. These findings indicate that the severe undernutrition associated with the eating disorder is the cause of the psychological changes.

Patient's perspective

From a mother of a daughter with anorexia nervosa:

'I feel so helpless and I cannot understand it. What she says is alien to common sense. She looks like my daughter but what comes out of her mouth is foreign. It is as though a stranger has taken over her mind.'

Two months later:

'I have my daughter back again. She looks and sounds like my daughter. There is still a along way to go. It is not over. She is eating and following the menu plan suggested by the hospital. She still makes no secret of her desire to be thinner but she says she will eat until after her exams.'

 Fact!

The brain of a patient with anorexia nervosa becomes smaller due to starvation.

These psychological changes are partly due to brain dehydration, as the brain actually becomes smaller, and partly due to changes in the chemicals in the brain at low weight. We do not currently fully understand the significance of these chemical changes, but they are important, as most are at an age when their brain is still maturing. Although patients with anorexia nervosa appear to revert to 'their old self' after weight gain, it has been suggested that some brain impairment may occur.

Psychological changes associated with anorexia nervosa

- Irritability

- Indecisiveness

- Poor concentration

- Confusion

- Depressed mood (feeling hopeless, guilty, worthless)

◆   Hyperactivity (feeling the need to keep busy)

◆   Insomnia

◆   Perfectionism

◆   Obsessive behaviour, particularly about food

◆   Withdrawal from people

Many anorexia nervosa sufferers are hyperactive and unable to relax. This is thought to be due to the low levels of the hormone leptin in their bloodstream (see page 45). This activity can be explained to patients as 'food-seeking behaviour' or foraging for food in times of famine. The hyperactivity may cause insomnia and early-morning waking in some sufferers.

A more unusual psychological disturbance is that anorexia nervosa (and bulimia nervosa) sufferers are more likely to shoplift than 'normal' eaters (see *Patient's perspective*: Debbie. In a study reported from the USA, one in three anorexia nervosa sufferers either shoplifted or stole, and many tended to self-harm. The reason for this psychological disturbance is unclear.

 Patient's perspective

Debbie was caught shoplifting two children's pillowcases and a box of chocolates. Ten days later she wrote:

'For the life of me I cannot believe why I did such a stupid and criminal act. Do I put it down to another destructive coping mechanism like that of anorexia and bulimia, which has been so familiar to me for the past 10 years? That is what I have to believe in order to come to terms with it and at the same time learn that I need to find other methods of coping with whatever pressures I may be under. The humiliation of that day and the repercussions are just not worth it. How could I explain to the lady who caught me what I was going through and that she should know that normally I just wouldn't do something like this? I actually tried but she told me that I was just the same as all the others and that it's a shame people like me don't go to jail. The silly thing is that I had more than enough money in my purse to pay for the things I'd taken and I think that only made things worse.

From then on, I think my body and mind relented to whatever was to happen and so as I was escorted from the shopping centre by two police officers, pushing my 21-month-old baby in her stroller, I convinced myself that people weren't staring at me and anyway this wasn't happening. Even at the police station, being questioned, fingerprinted, formally charged, and a court date given, I was oblivious to the reality of all that had happened and left the police station in a very dejected state, knowing that I had to explain all of this to my husband.'

Physical disturbances

The physical disturbances that affect anorexia nervosa sufferers are a consequence of the biochemical and hormonal changes and the loss of body fat (see box below). To conserve energy, the woman's heart rate slows, often only beating 40 times a minute. In spite of this, if she undertakes vigorous exercise, her heart rate increases, in a manner similar to that of 'normal' women. Her blood pressure is usually low. These two changes may lead to dizziness and occasionally fainting. The woman's skin may become dry and scaly, while soft, downy hair may develop on her face and body. Because she has very little fat beneath her skin, she loses her insulation. Her hands and feet feel cold and often look blue.

The lack of food and the biochemical changes lead to dilation of the intestines, slow movement of food through the gastrointestinal tract, and slow emptying of food from the stomach. All this gives the woman a feeling of being bloated and may aggravate constipation. Swelling of her feet and legs (oedema) may occur, particularly following attempts to gain weight by eating more food.

Psychological changes associated with anorexia nervosa

- Emaciation
- Slow heart beat (and pulse)
- Low blood pressure
- Bloating
- Constipation
- Swelling of hands and feet (oedema)

- Dry skin

- Appearance of fine facial and body hair (lanugo)

- Some loss of head hair

- Cold feet and hands

- Absent menstruation (amenorrhoea)

- Pale skin (mild anaemia)

Menstrual disturbances in anorexia nervosa

'I haven't had my periods for the last 10 years. I have forgotten that it is normal to have periods—and not normal to be without them. Even though it seems a lot easier and convenient for them to be non-existent, I'm also aware that I'm not experiencing the emotional state of a fully developed woman because of the shut-down of my hormonal system. I find that I am feeling deprived of this privilege but the only way to regain my periods is to do the positive thing that will remedy this situation—eat!'

 Fact!

A lack of menstrual periods reflects inadequate energy stored in the body for normal functioning.

Bleeding when taking the oral contraceptive does not indicate the presence of a normal menstrual cycle.

A major physical problem among females who have anorexia nervosa is that they fail to commence menstruation or their menstrual periods cease (amenorrhoea), often before much weight has been lost. This can remain undetected if the woman is taking oral contraception or other hormones. Some women believe that bleeding from the vagina when they are taking the oral contraceptive pill is menstruation. It is not—the bleeding occurs in response to the 'withdrawal' of the hormones in the pill during the pill-free week. This bleeding is referred to as 'withdrawal bleeding', and if the pill is taken as usually prescribed, this occurs every 4 weeks as there are 21 days of pills containing hormones followed by 7 days of no hormones.

The explanation of menstrual disturbances is rather complex, as it involves the interplay of a number of hormones. Control of these hormonal relationships takes place in an area of the brain called the hypothalamus, which in turn is influenced by messages from other parts of the brain and from the rest of the body. The hypothalamus orchestrates the changing patterns of release of follicle-stimulating hormone (FSH) and luteinizing hormone (LH) from the pituitary gland. These hormones are responsible for the production of the female hormones oestrogen and progesterone in the ovary and the events of the menstrual cycle: selection and growth of the egg (ovum) to be released at ovulation, ovulation, growth of the lining of the uterus (endometrium), and shedding of this lining (menstruation). This cycle of events is shown in Figure 7.2.

First menstruation (menarche) occurs when a woman has an adequate store of energy (as fat) in her body. The messenger informing the hypothalamus that the critical level of body fatness has been reached is the hormone leptin. When the body store of energy is low, the levels of leptin fall and the cells in the hypothalamus no longer stimulate the release of hormones to maintain the events of the menstrual cycle. The woman no longer ovulates and does not have her periods (amenorrhoea). In other words, her body returns to its prepubertal hormonal status where the levels of FSH, LH, oestrogen, and progesterone are all low and show little variation in their levels in the blood stream. It appears that the starved body responds by preventing conception of a baby where the mother would be unable to provide sufficient energy and nutrients for the fetus to survive the pregnancy.

 Fact!

Leptin reflects the amount of energy stored in the body.

Excessive exercise can also produce low body stores of energy and inhibit release of leptin with consequent amenorrhoea (see box below). A woman whose weight is below normal but is above the critical level, and who exercises excessively, such as a ballet dancer, may also fail to menstruate because she has inadequate energy stores in her body for her activity. Young athletes, if they become amenorrhoeic or if they have not commenced menstruating by 16, are advised to decrease their exercise and to increase their food intake so it is adequate for their activity levels.

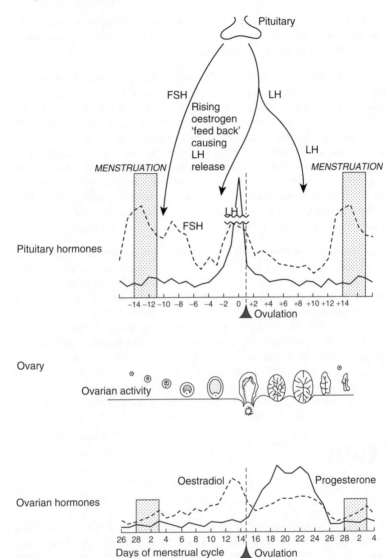

Figure 7.2 The control of menstruation. FSH, follicle-stimulating hormone; LH, Luteinizing hormone

Factors associated with amenorrhoea

◆ Low body weight/fat

◆ Large amount of weight lost (not at low weight)

◆ Excessive exercise

◆ Extreme weight-losing behaviours, e.g. vomiting

Return of menstruation

Once body weight increases above a critical level and adequate levels of leptin are produced, menstruation resumes, often after a delay. Menstruation usually starts again when the woman's body weight increases to reach a BMI of 17–19, but some women recommence menstruating at a lower body weight, particularly older women. Because of the uncertainty about when ovulation and menstruation will recommence, sexually active women who do not want to become pregnant (as babies born to women of low body weight have an increased chance of being underweight at birth) should not rely on lack of menstruation as protection against pregnancy. Some women have conceived while still at a low body weight and having had no periods for several years and no apparent weight change. For this reason, the woman or her partner should use a contraceptive method.

 Fact!

Amenorrhoea (no periods) is not a reliable form of contraception.

On the other hand, some women do not start menstruating again for some months, or even years, after returning to a normal body weight range. If a detailed history is taken from these women, it is usually found that they have been using weight-losing methods such as excessive exercise, self-induced vomiting, and laxative abuse, and in these cases the menstrual disturbance is almost certainly associated with the weight-losing behaviour (see box above). If this is not so, the woman should see her doctor and be assessed. A few women with irregular menses and overweight women may have polycystic ovarian syndrome.

Patient's perspective

Maria is the youngest daughter of a family who emigrated to Australia before she was born. At the age of 14, a year after her menstrual periods started, she became aware that her family were fat, and she did not want to become like them. Her weight was within the desirable range, a BMI of 20.6, and she was teased at school as being a 'sexy Italian'. She bought some slimming tablets from the chemist, but after taking them for 5 days stopped because they 'did no good'. As her friends at school were dieting, she decided to do so too. Her plan was to eat normally for 1 day and starve the next day. She tended to overeat when not starving so that after 2 months she had gained, not lost weight. She heard that if she took laxatives she would lose weight, and as her mother had given laxatives to the family when they had not opened their bowels, she felt she had 'permission' to use laxatives to lose weight. She also started exercising, spending 1 or 2 hours a day exercising, telling the family she was preparing for school sports.

Within a month of starting the exercise programme, her menstrual periods ceased, although she had only lost 2 kg (4 lbs). Maria was secretly pleased that she had no periods but was worried that people might know and wonder if she was normal. For the next 5 months, in spite of exercise and laxatives, her weight remained the same. In desperation to lose weight, Maria refused to eat with the family as the food was 'all pasta and unhealthy'. By the age of 16, she was dieting rigidly and was abusing laxatives. Her weight began to decrease and on her 18th birthday her BMI was 13.5. Her parents now intervened. She was admitted to hospital with a diagnosis of anorexia nervosa and started on a refeeding programme.

After 3 months, when she was discharged from hospital, her BMI was 21.3 and she had a menstrual period. At home, she continued to be afraid of becoming fat and returned to using excessive laxatives and dieted carefully to maintain a BMI of 19. She had no further menstrual periods until a year later when she found a job and a boyfriend of whom her parents approved. She ceased taking laxatives and started menstruating in spite of the fact that her weight had fallen and her BMI was 18.3.

Osteoporosis

A woman who does not menstruate regularly does not produce sufficient oestrogen to build up and maintain her peak bone density. For this reason, a young woman who has anorexia nervosa and whose periods have ceased for 6 months should have her bone mineral density measured and then monitored every 12 months.

Bone is continually being made and broken down. Oestrogen deficiency results in the new bone being formed and the high levels of cortisol from starvation means that existing bone is being reabsorbed more quickly. The net effect in patients with anorexia nervosa is a decrease in bone density and bone structure (called osteopenia for significant loss and osteoporosis for serious loss). In a woman who is of normal weight, is menstruating, and has sufficient calcium in her diet (1 g per day), her bones will reach their peak density when she is about 25. Provided her ovaries continue to produce oestrogen, her bones will remain at their peak density until she is 45.

 Fact!

Oral contraception is not a substitute for a woman's own hormones.

The woman can discuss taking a hormone replacement such as the contraceptive pill with her doctor, but recent research suggests that the benefits of oral contraception are small, even when calcium supplements are also taken. The less time women remain at a low body weight, the more modest the bone loss and the greater the chance of recovery to normal levels. Recovery of bone can take several years.

 Fact!

Treatment for osteoporosis is restoration and maintenance of normal body weight.

Sexuality

'Recovery means being interested in my husband sexually and not having to pretend.'

Coming to terms with one's sexuality is a major challenge facing adolescents. It appears that many women who have an eating disorder perceive an association between eating and their sexuality. Although women with anorexia nervosa show a wide range of sexual attitudes and behaviours, many avoid or withdraw from sexual activity when their eating disorder is active.

When people lose weight they report:

◆ losing their sexual feelings, often before menstruation ceases;

◆ a lack of lubrication of the vagina during sexual arousal; and

◆ discomfort during sexual intercourse.

These changes are caused by a decrease in the same hormones that are associated with the disturbance in menstruation. Some patients with anorexia nervosa report discomfort during gynaecological examination and avoid the use of tampons (for withdrawal bleeds when taking oral contraception). These women like to be in control of their bodies and are anxious about penetration; they are not more likely to have been sexually abused in the past than other women. During recovery, help with pelvic floor problems can make sexual activity more comfortable.

Women with a history of anorexia nervosa may have no experience of relationships and sexual activity, or they may simply experience boyfriends, marriage, and children at a later age.

Marriage and children

Compared with women who do not have an eating disorder, anorexia nervosa patients after treatment are twice as likely to live alone and not to marry. If they do marry, they are twice as likely to remain childless. This may be changing as more women are seeking assisted conception, e.g. *in vitro* fertilization.

8

Treatment and outcome of anorexia nervosa and anorexia nervosa-like disorders

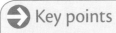 Key points

- Over a period of 1–5 years, most patients recover from anorexia nervosa; most relapses occur in the first year after treatment, usually when there are stressful situations

- Treatment involves refeeding back to the normal body mass index (BMI) range, establishing 'normal' eating behaviour, and ceasing weight-losing behaviour

- Treatment involves supportive psychotherapy and a range of psychological therapies and techniques that help the woman manage her eating-disordered thoughts and her moods while achieving the treatment aims

- Ongoing psychological treatment helps her cope with stress, anxiety, and dysphoric moods without using food and eating-disordered behaviour

- Most patients with anorexia nervosa are treated in hospital at least once during their illness, needing the supervision and containment provided and access to a multidisciplinary team of experienced professionals

- A graduated exercise programme should be implemented during treatment

'Although it has been a slow and painful process, I have finally reached the once "unattainable" recovery that I thought you only read about in books. One by one, the ridiculous rituals and lists of rules I had set for myself (in order to control my body and life) were literally crossed out. From never using moisturisers on my body (for fear that the fats would seep through my skin) to overloading foods with chilli, I gradually learned to let go of these habits and ironically found I was getting a greater sense of control over myself.'

Aims of treatment

The aims of the treatment of anorexia nervosa are listed in the box below.

Aims of treatment of anorexia nervosa

◆ To help the woman increase her weight by refeeding, so that it lies between a BMI of 19 and 25

◆ To establish normal eating behaviour, emphasizing structured eating and regular eating episodes

◆ To help her acquire helpful attitudes to food and eating, and be flexible in her food choices

◆ To help her decrease her preoccupation with thoughts of food, eating, and her body

◆ To help her gain feelings of control over her eating, body, and exercise without her eating-disordered behaviour

◆ To help her stop using behaviours aimed at weight loss, including excessive exercise

◆ To explain the physical and psychological symptoms she may experience during treatment

◆ To address problems such as relationships or family problems that may prevent recovery

◆ To help her cope with unpleasant feelings without resorting to disordered eating and weight loss

◆ To provide support and reassurance

Before any treatment is offered, the doctor makes a careful physical examination and may order some laboratory tests (see Chapter 5). The therapist must have taken a careful history to confirm that the woman has anorexia nervosa and that her body weight is not low as a consequence of experimenting with dieting, her choice of career, drugs, her lifestyle, or another illness. The importance of distinguishing between women who have anorexia nervosa and women who maintain a low body weight for other reasons is shown by Zoe's story (see *Patient's perspective*).

 Patient's perspective

Zoe had always wanted to be a ballet dancer, and at the age of 15 she applied for a place in a prestigious full-time ballet school. Her teacher had impressed on her the need to be thin. Zoe said she had never had to control her weight as she went to ballet classes three evenings each week and didn't eat between school and the class. Six months before the selection process, her ballet teacher told her that she would have to lose some weight or she would not be selected. At that time, her BMI was 18.5.

She started dieting and soon her weight loss was noticed by the headmistress of her school, who contacted Zoe's mother, fearing that Zoe had anorexia nervosa. Her mother at once took Zoe to a doctor who arranged for her to be admitted to hospital for refeeding. Her BMI was now 16. In hospital, she refused to eat or gave her food to other patients. She adopted this strategy because she believed that if she gained weight her chance of selection to the ballet school would be jeopardized. Her resistance to refeeding confirmed to the health professionals that Zoe had anorexia nervosa. She was also considered by them to be uncooperative, untruthful, and difficult.

When we talked to Zoe, her fear of not being selected for the ballet school became clear. We reassured her that, in Australia, young ballet dancers needed to have a BMI of at least 18 or they would not 'look good on stage'. Zoe accepted the reassurance and gained weight in the next 5 weeks. She was selected to train at the ballet school and has maintained her weight within the range acceptable for a dancer since that time. She does not appear to be more preoccupied with food, dieting, or her weight than the other ballet students and is enjoying the training at which she has been very successful.

The reverse situation to that of Zoe's can also occur, when the diagnosis of anorexia nervosa may be more difficult, as many young women who have the disorder initially deny that they have any problems and believe they can change their behaviour if they choose.

Psychological management

Anorexia nervosa is a psychosomatic disorder, during which psychological and physical symptoms develop because of self-induced starvation and other methods of inducing weight loss. The mood of many patients improves when they are eating an adequate amount of food to ensure that their bodies are no longer nutritionally deprived.

 Fact!

Psychological treatment is of limited use without weight gain.

At very low body weight, patients may find it difficult to concentrate and impossible to use some of the psychological strategies employed in the treatment of eating disorders (see Chapter 6). The main treatment is individual supportive psychotherapy and includes:

◆ acceptance of an appropriate menu plan;

◆ acceptance of regular adjustment of the menu plan;

◆ monitoring of weight and behaviour;

◆ monitoring of moods, thoughts, and feelings;

◆ food and nutritional information, challenging the unhelpful beliefs;

◆ counselling about eating and potentially dangerous methods of losing weight;

◆ involving the family or partner as appropriate; and

◆ helping her to find other ways of coping with unpleasant feelings.

Many psychological therapies and techniques ranging from distraction to mindfulness can be employed depending on the age of the person, their degree of emaciation, the length of their illness, and their personality and resilience. Cognitive, behavioural, and motivational techniques are employed, and interaction with other patients and with recovered sufferers can be reassuring and supportive. A summary of commonly used psychological therapies is given on pages 97–9.

Psychological changes may be slow, and, early in the treatment, sufferers and their families may wonder whether psychological treatment is effective. Over a longer time period, sometimes as long as 2–5 years, unhelpful and destructive attitudes about eating and body image are slowly replaced by constructive and positive thoughts, and what were anxiety-producing situations are accepted without concern.

The following suggestions are some simple tasks that help the woman to realize she can: (1) recognize and 'fight' her disordered thoughts; (2) accept them and choose to ignore them; and (3) gain insight into the associations of mood, food, and weight. Parents also help if they say they will not talk to the 'eating disorder' but want to talk to their daughter. Annoying as it may seem to the sufferer at the time, this helps everyone.

Suggestions:

List the thoughts and behaviours you have that belong to your eating disorder.

Write a letter to your eating disorder saying what you like about it and what you don't.

Write a letter saying goodbye to your eating disorder.

Keep a daily diary of your thoughts and moods.

 Patient's perspective

The following was written by a patient, Stephanie, in response to a task set by her dietician/psychologist. Stephanie was asked if she would like to compare the promises her illness had made to her with what had occurred in reality. She wrote:

The labyrinth

Promise: Order and satisfaction in your life. *Reality*: Disappointment and depression.

Promise: Discipline and control. *Reality*: Confusion and uncertainty.

Promise: Popularity and sociability. *Reality*: Isolation and loneliness.

Promise: Respect and admiration. *Reality*: Pity.

Promise: Perfection in all areas of life. *Reality*: Physical and mental self-destruction.

Anorexia is a labyrinth of lies and destruction. No matter what options or solutions it may offer to you, every choice will ultimately end in sadness and solitude. It works in the utmost deceiving and almost undetectable ways burying your true personality nearly to the point that even you may find it hard to recognize that once happy, vibrant person you were and still can be. The truth and reality I have learned is that its power is merely an illusion. I simply had to believe I was stronger and gradually dig up those characteristics that represent me as a confident and content individual, buried beneath the lies of anorexia. Often it's hard to believe I have it in me to fight because again and again anorexia tells me I have nothing to fight for that is worthy enough to save from destruction. But this is where I have to pay careful attention to the people around me, making a conscious effort to listen, believe, and most importantly 'remember' (not dismiss) compliments and virtues they claim they saw and still see in me (despite anorexia's efforts to bury them!).

Anorexia creates its rituals through obsession and fear. The trick is to untrain these as rapidly as it trains. In the beginning, it was an effort to force myself to ignore anorexia and create new habits—but if I listened to my heart, friends, and family, they always guided me whenever I questioned my actions.

You are able to train yourself back into reality and normality no matter how unattainable it may seem at the time. Whenever I feel myself weakening in the fight and hear anorexia's criticisms polluting my mind, I hold on to memories of the past—how I was liked, happy, relaxed, and content—and I work on regaining these attributes. No one and certainly no disease of any kind has the power to change or destroy your memories of the past—so this is my power that anorexia cannot touch.

Rather than fighting the thoughts in my mind, which tends to be confusing and a no win situation, I have learned to fight 'Anorexia'. I question its answers, disobey its orders, knowing it's evil. Destroy it before it can destroy you and win the fight—I think this is truly an opportunity to achieve something many will never even begin to understand.

Family therapy

Family therapy that assists a patient's family in fighting the eating disorder can be the treatment of choice for very young patients with motivated families. The therapist first assesses the family and explores the family dynamics, and then supports them by helping them to manage the young person at home. This involves the family preparing the food and supervising each meal and snack the child must eat. This can be difficult if both parents are working and in families with a sole parent, as it can be very intensive—each eating episode can take hours rather than minutes. This approach is less effective as patients become older, but is used after a person has been treated in hospital and has learnt to eat and follow an adequate menu plan. By this stage, young women are usually able to return to school or work and to cope with minimal supervision of lunchtime eating. Some general advice from a parent with experience of family therapy and family support therapy and with years of coping with living with a daughter with anorexia nervosa is given in the box below.

Tips from a parent

- ◆ Fight the illness, not the person

- ◆ Don't blame yourself for causing the illness

- ◆ Get professional help as quickly as possible

- ◆ Try to normalize family life

- ◆ Educate yourself about the illness

- ◆ Give unconditional love and support

- ◆ Try not to be too secretive about the illness

- ◆ Try to keep your sense of humour

- ◆ Give respect to the person with the illness

- ◆ Be firm when necessary

Where should a woman with anorexia nervosa be treated?

Young anorexia nervosa sufferers who have only recently lost weight and whose BMI is greater than 16 can be treated by their family doctor or therapist together with a dietician. This combination of health professionals provides the expertise to help the majority of young women who have problems associated with strict dieting and the consequent weight loss. If she does not quickly respond to this initial intervention by changing her eating behaviours and beginning to increase her weight, more specialized help is indicated. This may involve her attending a specialized eating-disorder service as a day-patient or as an inpatient in hospital and receiving treatment by a multidisciplinary team of professionals (see pages 92–3). The indications for admission to hospital are given in the box below.

 Fact!

Most women with anorexia nervosa are treated in hospital at some time during their illness.

Day-patient treatment allows the woman to live at home while attending a specialized eating-disorder unit where she receives help to make the changes needed for her recovery. Her daily (usually 3–5 days a week) attendance at the eating-disorder unit gives her access to a team of supportive and experienced people who can help her cope with the range of problems she experiences. She will have individual sessions and group sessions, educating her and teaching her psychological strategies. In hospital, treatment occurs every day and patients are usually encouraged to continue with their studies if they wish.

Indications for admission to hospital

- ◆ Lack of response to outpatient treatment

- ◆ Living too far from outpatient or day-patient treatment

- ◆ Very low body weight with life-threatening physiological changes

- ◆ Serious cardiac and electrolyte disturbances

- ◆ A need to separate the patient from family problems

- ◆ Possible risk of suicide or self-harm

- ◆ Lack of support outside hospital

- ◆ The family need rest and time for recuperation

- ◆ The woman prefers to be an inpatient

Increasing body weight

Although anorexia nervosa is a psychosomatic problem, the first priority in treatment must be to achieve weight gain. The long-term aim is for the woman to learn to increase her weight and to maintain it within the normal desirable range for her age and height (BMI of 19–25). A BMI of 19 is the minimum weight for normal physiological function.

Refeeding

Refeeding is the main way in which a sufferer is helped to gain weight. During the refeeding programme, she is provided with a menu plan and with nutritional information by her dietician, so that she can learn to eat normally, with three meals and three snacks each day at regular times. Eating episodes are supervised by a dietician, psychologist, or specialist nurse, and eating within acceptable time limits is encouraged. Each patient is encouraged to gradually take more and more responsibility for her own eating until she no longer requires any supervision. Normal eating is described in Chapter 10.

Weighing

Because minor daily changes in weight occur and because of the patient's preoccupation with her weight, it is preferable to weigh the patient two or three times a week, rather than daily. Weighing has to be done carefully and the nurse must make sure that the patient does not cheat, for example, by drinking water just before being weighed or by putting weights in her pockets (see box below). Occasional weighing at unpredictable times is used to check if the patient is cheating.

Methods of cheating to increase weight

- Drink large amounts of water the night before being weighed
- Avoid emptying the bladder before being weighed
- Drink bath or shower water
- Binge eat the night before
- Wear heavy jewellery or heavy clothing (such as ski braces)
- Sew or insert weights into clothes before being weighed

Menu plan

During the refeeding programme, the woman is expected to eat a varied diet that is balanced in macronutrients and micronutrients, with the inclusion of 'feared' high-energy foods in moderation. The aim is for a weight increase of 1.0–1.5 kg (2–3 lb) a week if she is in hospital and 0.3–0.5 (0.5–1 lb) a week if she is an outpatient.

 Fact!

A woman can be believed, but an eating disorder cannot be truthful.

In the early stages of refeeding, this weight increase can be achieved with a smaller amount of 'normal' food providing 6700–7700 kJ (1600–1800 kcal) a day, depending on the patient's previous nutritional intake. Once the woman can eat this quantity of food without vomiting or overexercising, increases in food intake will be necessary. This should be discussed between the patient and her dietician at least once a week.

Complying with eating the amount of food recommended, particularly in the first few weeks, is extremely difficult for each woman. Patients are terrified their weight will increase rapidly and not stop, even if they eat normally. During this time, they are likely to try to choose low-energy foods and to cheat in the amount they eat. Some of the ways they try to avoid eating are given in the box below.

Methods of cheating with the menu plan

◆ Hide food in table napkins or tissues

◆ Leave the crust of toast or bread on the plate, discarding the rest

◆ Dispose of food into pockets, shoes, bras, stuffed toys, cupboards, or out of the window

◆ Keep food in the mouth and discard it when cleaning the teeth

◆ Surreptitiously feed the family dog under the table

◆ Keep high-energy food under long fingernails and wash hands after eating

◆ Dilute milk, juice, or a high-energy supplement with water

◆ Puncture drink cartons so the milk, juice, or high energy supplement leaks out before it is drunk

If the woman feels that the amount of food is too large and too bulky—usually if it contains more than 12,600 kJ (3000 kcal)—then high-energy drinks or food supplements may be used. Some women need to increase their food intake to 12,600–20,000 kJ (3000–5000 kcal) a day to reach their target weight. Once this has been reached, a menu providing a maintenance intake of 10,000–11,000 kJ (2000–2400 kcal) a day is constructed.

Bedrest

If the woman does not respond, a more structured programme, involving her resting on her bed and using a wheelchair when necessary, can be implemented for a short time. The aim is to give her the supervision and containment necessary to allow a small amount of weight to be gained and for her nutrition to improve. Although this appears to be a very strict programme, women who are at very low body weight are frequently unable to think clearly and the fear of gaining weight is overpowering.

Nasogastric feeding

Nasogastric or tube feeding is another method of refeeding. This involves passing a thin, flexible tube into the stomach by way of the nose and oesophagus, through which measured amounts of liquid food can be given three or four times a day. The tube must be introduced by an experienced person and the patient must be monitored carefully in a medical setting throughout the early refeeding period. This method is not without complications—the patient may retain too much fluid, and if feeding is too rapid, 'refeeding syndrome' may occur (page 137). The patient's fluid, weight, and electrolytes must be monitored. She may also try to remove, destroy, or block the tube.

Some patients who accept they have a problem but feel unable to eat view nasogastric feeding very positively. They may express relief that the responsibility for eating has been taken away from them. As they gain weight, the intensity of their fears of eating decrease and they are able to start to eat again.

Advantages and disadvantages of nasogastric feeding

Advantages

- Can be used if the patient refuses treatment

- The woman can feel she is not responsible for her weight gain

---

◆ Less time is usually spent at a low weight

◆ Less time is usually spent in hospital, so it is less expensive, and there is less time away from school, work, family, and friends

Disadvantages

◆ Does not teach 'normal' eating behaviour

◆ The woman does not take responsibility for her own eating

◆ She does not learn how much to eat or drink

◆ Patients can still find ways to avoid weight gain

Refusal to gain weight

Some women are unable to recognize they are ill and may refuse treatment. At a very low weight, a woman may not be able to make an informed decision about her treatment. Patients with anorexia nervosa can be very convincing in their arguments, particularly those involving weight gain, and they will agree to anything that will delay weight gain and will disagree with any suggestions that involve immediate treatment. They may even choose death over a life of constant vigilance against weight gain. These attitudes change as weight is gained and patients respond to adequate nutrition. When parents and doctors consider a patient is sufficiently impaired and unable to make an informed decision about accepting treatment, nasogastric feeding may be necessary.

Physical effects of refeeding

When refeeding begins, there is the possibility of a rapid weight gain, which results from the expansion of fluid in the tissues between the body cells (the extracellular compartment) and an increase in the body's glycogen–water pool (see page 201). This may cause great anxiety and the woman needs to be assured that the weight gain, which is due to rehydration, will resolve spontaneously if she continues to adhere to the refeeding programme.

Suggestion: Stand on the scales so you cannot see your weight; ask not to be told.

Suggestion: Do not buy new, close-fitting clothes during refeeding.

The other potentially dangerous complication is the occurrence of the 'refeeding syndrome'. The patient should always be monitored carefully in the early stages of refeeding, as when this syndrome occurs, among other biochemical changes, much of the phosphorus in the blood is taken into the body cells leading to a low level of blood phosphate (hypophosphataemia). Death may occur unless phosphorus supplements are given. Although this occurs rarely, the people who are most at risk are those who are:

◆ extremely emaciated;

◆ have been starving; or

◆ have been vomiting or abusing laxatives.

Establishing normal eating behaviour

Suggestion: List the foods you avoid eating, from most to least scary.
Suggestion: List the places you avoid going and the people you avoid eating around.
Suggestion: Make a plan to challenge your eating-related fears one by one.

'Normal eating' involves more than eating sufficiently to gain weight. Most patients with anorexia nervosa restrict the number of different foods they eat, so the second aim of treatment is for the patient to learn to:

◆ choose from a wide range of foods to provide her body with the nutrients it needs;

◆ eat all foods in sensible amounts;

◆ eat in front of people she knows and does not know;

◆ eat at different venues, restaurants, food halls, and coffee shops, and at home, school, or work;

◆ eat and be comfortable eating in social situations;

◆ understand how much she can eat without weight gain; and

◆ develop 'normal' eating behaviours (see Chapter 10).

These matters are explored and discussed during the refeeding programme. Many eating-disorder experts believe that this 'psycho-education' is most effective if conducted with a group of patients. All of the challenges listed above should be achieved during refeeding.

Suggestion: Make a list of the challenges you need to confront and mark them off as each is successfully accomplished.

Ceasing weight-losing behaviours

Patients find reassurance on learning what effects to expect when they stop vomiting and using laxatives. These are described in detail in Chapter 10. The commonest symptoms are:

◆ an initial weight gain due to rehydration;

◆ abdominal bloating;

◆ abdominal discomfort or cramps (hot packs can be used for these); and

◆ constipation or irritable bowel symptoms, which may persist for some time.

As the patients are preoccupied with their body weight and abdominal fullness, these are the very symptoms that make them anxious and may induce them to return to vomiting and laxatives unless they know that these symptoms are to be expected.

The place of exercise during treatment

 Fact!

A graduated exercise programme is part of the treatment plan.

Hyperactivity and agitation occur during exercise withdrawal.

It is sensible for an anorexia nervosa patient, if she so wishes, to embark on a graduated exercise programme while under treatment, so that she may learn and accept a sensible exercise programme that is appropriate for her and which aims to achieve the levels of exercise she is likely to do after weight gain. If the woman is not gaining weight while being refed, the amount of exercise she does must be reduced or may have to stop. Studies have shown that women who have anorexia nervosa gain weight faster if their activity is limited during treatment.

The reasons for including graduated exercise during treatment are:

◆ to feel better about themselves and their body;

◆ to learn or relearn what 'normal activity' and 'sensible exercise' consist of;

- to reduce the size of the abdomen by redistributing fat and increasing intestinal tone during refeeding;

- to increase the recovery of lean body mass by increasing the muscle mass during refeeding;

- to provide some relief for the low weight-induced hyperactivity of some patients;

- to provide some relief for the agitation of patients 'withdrawing' from excessive exercise;

- to prevent the secret exercising that some patients feel compelled to do;

- to prevent the replacement of the eating disorder by exercise disorder (see page 31 and *Patient's perspective* below).

 Patient's perspective

'There's no question about it, it has to be done. It's like I can't see beyond the actual obsession. I can't do anything to distract myself. I wouldn't know what to do till I'd done it. I just hurry and get it over and done with as fast as possible so I can relax. It's like a duty I have to perform before I can continue with life. The stairs are the worst—I only do it at night, although the thought pops into my head every time I have to walk up or down them. It is at night when everyone is home, so I have to pick my time and walk softly. I feel everyone else is controlling when I can do it, trying to stop me. Just leave me alone and let me finish. I have to get it done! I can't live, I don't know how to live without them. If I don't do it I will be a self-indulgent, lazy slob. When I'm tired, my thoughts are fuzzy, so I can't figure them out; when I'm alert I have enough energy to run across the Nullabor. Let me do them, get it over and done with, put it behind me, let it be over for another night. Quickly, quickly, faster and faster. Sometimes I feel so ashamed of myself for doing this—I just close my eyes or focus on how good it will be when it's all over. It's so lovely. My awareness is heightened, I can hear everything and feel everything and gosh, it hurts.'

Medications

 Fact!

Food is the best oral medication.

Antidepressants

Medications play an insignificant part in the management of anorexia nervosa. If an antidepressant drug is needed, one of the selective serotonin reuptake inhibitors (SSRIs), such as fluoxetine or paroxetine, is preferred. These drugs are very effective for women who are depressed and who suffer from obsessive–compulsive disorder (OCD), but the results from recent studies of their use in the treatment of women suffering with anorexia nervosa, both during and after weight gain, have been disappointing.

Antipsychotics

When very low weight patients with anorexia nervosa find it impossible to accept help to eat sufficiently to achieve weight gain, very low doses of a novel antipsychotic drug, such as olanzapine, can help. Patients have reported that their disordered thoughts are less intense and are 'slowed down' so that they can make decisions about their treatment. They are also observed to be less agitated and restless. Once body weight is increasing and adequate nutrition is restored, the medication can be ceased. Because these drugs are known to stimulate appetite in some patients with psychotic illnesses, patients with eating disorders are fearful of this occurring. Patients need reassurance that the dose being prescribed is very small and that at these doses appetite is not stimulated. It is helpful if they can talk to other patients who have taken them.

Relapses and relapse prevention

In the first year after treatment, 20–30% of patients with anorexia nervosa who have apparently recovered start to lose weight again and relapse. If the woman can maintain her body weight in the normal range for a year, there is less likelihood of relapse, although it may still occur. Later relapses usually occur at times of stress, when the woman feels helpless to change what is happening in her life. Women are most likely to relapse if:

◆ they were severely ill and needed treatment in hospital;

◆ they maintained a body weight just below the normal range;

- they kept rigid, controlled eating and exercise patterns;

- they have other medical or psychiatric problems such as diabetes or depression;

- they have swapped their eating disorder for another problem such as exercise disorder, or use of drugs or alcohol;

- they are less resilient in stressful circumstances.

As well as being able to contact their therapist easily and quickly, in many cases the relapse can be prevented if the woman follows the guidelines outlined in the box below.

Relapse prevention guidelines

To prevent relapse, the woman should:

- Allow her body weight to increase a little after she has achieved the target recommended during refeeding. This permits her body to correct the ratio of lean (mostly muscle) tissue to fat tissue so that its composition is normal.

- Try to avoid any further weight loss for any reason. For example, if she is ill and loses weight, she should try to regain that weight (no matter how little) as quickly as possible.

- Avoid situations that keep her thinking about food, her body shape, her weight, or exercise. For this reason, she should avoid working in a job that is around food or in a gym or fitness centre.

- Avoid changing her routine too much.

- Avoid long holidays or trips overseas. In an unfamiliar environment, with the loss of routine, frequent new experiences, and different foods, she may feel that she has lost control and revert to old behaviours to cope.

- Find ways of coping with stress and unpleasant feelings without resorting to control of weight, eating, or exercise.

- Learn the early warning signs of relapse and seek help as soon as possible before weight is lost.

- Maintain contact with her therapist.

Patient's perspective

Kara, a 22-year-old ex-patient, returned from overseas and entered the eating-disorders unit for refeeding. Her story is an example of what may happen if a woman who is recovering from anorexia nervosa goes overseas before she is fully recovered:

'I had been looking forward to the trip for months, but when I arrived at the airport the reality of going finally hit me ... and I found myself asking, "What am I doing?" I didn't know what to expect and it was the first time I'd left home and been so far away from my parents. Plus, my eating wasn't all that stable, although I tried to ignore that fact. In the plane, I was already "cutting back", as I wasn't flexible enough to cope with the type of meals that were served, and as we changed time zones a few times, it seemed like I was faced with dinner when it theoretically should have been about 3 o'clock in the morning! As I was settling into a new life, I was always looking in the shops for the types of food I was used to eating at home and felt safe with. I became aware that I was trying to take Australia with me, and found it difficult to accept a different culture and cuisine, due to the rigidity of my habitual daily intake.

As it was winter, we ate a lot of heavy foods, such as potatoes with creamy sauces, fatty meats, and greasy vegetables. This, as well as the custom of eating the main meal in the middle of the day, was guilty and anxiety-producing for me, as I kept thinking of my meal sitting here in my stomach the whole afternoon. To combat this, I often went for a bike ride or to the local swimming pool. I tried to occupy myself as much as possible with study, writing letters, and going out, so that I wouldn't be reminded that I was hungry or have an excuse to eat. I was also doing exercises every night in my room—an obsession which had started many months ago at home.

As a result of excessive exercise and eating as little as I could get away with, I kept losing weight. I also began isolating myself in my room, and feeling very lonely and depressed. I kept longing for the security of home, and became increasingly withdrawn and secretive, bottling up my emotions inside and believing no one could possibly understand.

By this stage I was so caught up in my own thoughts that I could see no other way but down. It was like my eating disorder was ruling me again, and I was made aware of how powerful it is.

When I look back on it now, I realize how important it is to be honest with yourself when planning big changes in your life. I would not recommend that anyone who has or has had an eating disorder go overseas unless she is completely recovered, and has the strength to recognize her "triggers" and instigate appropriate coping strategies. Adapting to a new situation and lifestyle without the "policemen"—that is, family, friends, and doctors—can be stressful. The easiest and most natural thing to do is to resort to old coping mechanisms and behaviours, which can ultimately be destructive. The prospect of an overseas trip is of course very exciting and challenging, but you can't fit your eating disorder in your suitcase too.'

Outcome of anorexia nervosa

Statistics

Between 50% and 80% of patients with anorexia nervosa completely or partially recover after treatment lasting 6 months to 6 years. Approximately 40–50% of sufferers will recover completely, and 30–40% recover sufficiently to lead a normal life, although they may continue to have thoughts or behaviours they associate with an eating disorder. These thoughts are described by patients as 'always there but the volume is turned down', 'they come and go', or 'they can be ignored'. It is hard to know whether these thoughts differ from those of women in the community who do not have an eating disorder. The important thing is the woman has a good quality of life.

Recovery is more likely if:

◆ the woman is younger, not at very low weight, not overweight previously;

◆ it is the first time she has received treatment and treatment is started early;

◆ the woman's family is supportive, and there is no conflict among family members;

◆ she is a 'dieter and exerciser' rather than a 'vomiter and purger';

◆ her anorexia nervosa is not associated with bulimia nervosa.

Many women who have apparently recovered may continue to need support.

Patient's perspective

Kylie had four admissions to hospital for refeeding. Before and after being discharged from hospital for the fourth time she wrote to her doctor:

'I know that I still look too thin, but I just don't seem able to regain the weight I lost in the last four months. It may be because I left home then. I was very worried about how I'd cope when I started living away from home again, and tried to be strict with myself about "cutting back" on food. I don't think I did "cut back", but I suppose I'm a lot more active now at work than I was when I was at home leading a life of (enforced) leisure. However, I find it almost impossible to let myself eat more. As you may remember, my problem has always been an "eating-food" one, rather than a concern with weight. Basically, I still think the same way as I have for a long time, and I don't suppose this will ever change.'

A year after her fourth admission, Kylie wrote again:

'Considering everything, I've been keeping quite well. I've maintained my weight since I left the clinic (over a year ago now!) though I haven't put any more on. I'm still not overconfident about how I would cope on my own, i.e. if I was preparing and responsible for all my own food. So many of the old attitudes are still lying dormant and I have to be ever-vigilant that they don't exert too much influence. All in all, it's still not terribly easy, though I must admit that I do think less and less about being an "anorexic".'

Approximately 15–25% of patients continue to suffer from anorexia nervosa, requiring intermittent therapy over many years.

Mortality

Death due to anorexia nervosa gets newspaper headlines, particularly if the victim is a celebrity. However, less than 3% of patients die from the effects of the eating disorder (half of whom die following a drug overdose). In short-term studies, predominantly of adolescent women, the death rate is 0–2%. Long-term studies that include the 20% of chronic anorexia nervosa sufferers suggest that up to 6% of these patients will die over a period of years. With our greater community awareness about anorexia nervosa, victims can receive help earlier in their illness, and with more professionals trained to manage the illness, the death rate is likely to be lower in the next decade.

A good outcome

 Fact!

Refeeding, re-education about eating habits, and explanation of physical symptoms are only initial goals in the treatment.

Treatment must include helping the woman to gain insight into her thoughts and behaviours and find other, gentler ways to cope with anxiety and unpleasant moods without succumbing to an eating disorder (see *Patient's perspective*).

 Patient's perspective

'While I thought anorexia was a way of gaining more control over my life, I know now it did completely the opposite. I have never felt so clear about my goals, so in control of my body, emotions, and path in life than I do today—a recovered anorexic.

I still occasionally weaken and the perfectionist in me comes out. I have realized it is normally when my life gets a little stressful, or big changes are occurring around me. But this is when I reach out to close family and friends who know my history and who are able to offer support and help keep things in perspective. I do everything possible to keep from reaching out to old eating-disorder habits for this feeling of comfort.

It is by no means easy, but it is possible. It is a retraining of the mind and body, undoing old habits and most importantly recognizing the times I am vulnerable, acknowledging why I feel this way and accepting that it is okay to feel stressed or overwhelmed at times. My trick is not going through these stages or trying to deal with them alone, in fear of using food to control my situation.

I consciously choose alternatives. The most effective way I have found is trying to reduce pressures and responsibilities a little while I am going through a stressful period rather than trying to be the "perfect" wife, employee, friend, etc. I am honest with those around me and ask for help for that period of time, such as asking my husband to help out a bit more around the house, asking for some assistance with projects at work, asking my friends for advice, and seeing a bit more of my mum and dad for dinners during the week.

> Basically, I am looking out for and protecting myself as if I am my own best friend.'

One patient described what her recovery meant to her as follows:

- Being able to go out to breakfast, lunch, or dinner, and not having to worry about the exact time I eat my meal, or what others around me are eating, and happily choosing what I feel like on the menu rather than the lowest in fat.

- Having more time for my friends and family rather than having to spend so much time on keeping food diaries, calculating calories, obsessing about my weight, and punishing myself.

- Feeling happy and relaxed, not wound up, on the brink of tears, or at breaking point every minute.

- Not having to be at the gym at exactly the right time to start a workout.

- Regaining lost memories that anorexia deleted from my life through starvation.

- Not being so short-tempered and having fewer fights with people.

- Being able to handle stress at work.

- Having increased concentration and motivation.

- Feeling like a woman.

- Not obsessing over meaningless/careless comments made about food, my appearance, my weight, or my body by strangers.

- Being able to control my own moods and emotions and not rely on other people's judgements of me to feel good or bad. It means having my own opinion.

- No more guilt or the lies anorexia encouraged me to tell my closest relatives.

A summary of the treament of anorexia nervosa is shown in Figure 8.1.

Summary of the treatment of anorexia nervosa

* Clinically not seriously ill
* Previous hospital treatment.

* Severely ill on clinical examination
* Failure of outpatient or day-patient treatment
* The woman expresses a preference

↓

Evaluate physical and biochemical status

↓   ↓

Usually treat as an outpatient or as day patient

Other suggestions and support to help patient:
* increase weight slowly by 0.3–0.5 kg (0.5–1 lb) a week
* stop using weight-losing behaviour
* learn sensible eating patterns

Usually admit to hospital

Provide a programme to help the patient:
* increase weight by 1–1.5 kg (2–3 lbs) a week
* cease weight-losing behaviour
* learn sensible eating patterns
* exercise appropriately for body weight

↓

If the above goals are not achieved, usually admit to hospital

Throughout the programme provide:
* supportive psychotherapy
* psychological therapies
* help for other perceived problems (marital, family, medical)
* help establishing structured eating patterns appropriate to lifestyle and age
* help in developing sensible exercise patterns
* confidence in ability to eat sensibly

Later, provide help for the patient:
* to stabilize weight in the desirable range
* to continue to avoid dangerous weight-losing methods
* to decrease preoccupation with weight and food
* to improve self-esteem so that it no longer depends on her body and shape

↓

The overall aim is to help the patient:
* to live a normal life
* to be able to cope with problems and challenges

9

Bulimia nervosa and bulimia nervosa-like disorders

→ Key points

* Binge eating is an episode of eating that the person feels is out of their control, that they cannot stop, and where they consume an inappropriately large amount of food

* The food consumed during a binge is very varied in content and amount, and contains foods people will not allow themselves to eat at other times

* Patients with bulimia nervosa use extreme methods of weight control: most induce vomiting, some exercise excessively, and some drastically reduce their food intake between binges

* Binge eating is precipitated by anxious and dysphoric moods, which are relieved by binge eating; vomiting may be more efficient at relieving these unpleasant feelings

* Bulimia nervosa, anorexia nervosa, and binge-eating disorder have many similar features and people can fulfil the diagnostic criteria for more than one at different times

* The incidence of bulimia nervosa is 1–3% and for bulimia-like disorders may be as high as 6–8%

'I think that I look forward to a binge-eating session. Exactly what I am thinking is vague, but on reflection it is: "Oh good, I won't have to think about dieting any more—what a relief." If anything happens which delays the start of the binge, I become quite angry and rather rude to the person who caused the delay. This anger is not warranted and is totally inappropriate—it could be likened to a temper tantrum.'

Description

Anorexia nervosa and bulimia nervosa have many features in common (see Chapter 2). The diagnosis of anorexia nervosa is made if the woman who is binge eating and using extreme methods of weight loss is at low body weight, while a diagnosis of bulimia nervosa is made when she is at higher weight, although there may have been no other change in the features of her illness. The difference between bulimia nervosa and binge-eating disorder is the presence of inappropriate weight-losing behaviours and hence a high body weight. The definition and diagnostic criteria for bulimia nervosa and binge-eating disorder are given in Chapter 2.

Demographics

The demographics of bulimia nervosa and binge-eating disorder are given in the box below. The true prevalences may be higher, as only those women who seek medical help are identifiable. Many do not tell their doctor about their eating habits, mistakenly believing that *only* people who induce vomiting have bulimia, and, as a result, they are often investigated for gastrointestinal problems, such as irritable bowel syndrome, or gynaecological problems, such as infertility and menstrual disturbances, or are thought to be depressed and are given antidepressants. Binge eating in response to food restriction can occur in children, when parents who are attempting to keep their children 'healthy' and prevent them becoming overweight do not provide sufficient energy for their growth, development, and energy expenditure. Men and women of all ages will seek help for obesity but not for binge eating.

The demographics of bulimia nervosa

◆ Life-time prevalence of bulimia nervosa is 1–3%

◆ Predominately occurs in post-pubertal women

- Peak incidence is at 18–25 years

- Onset usually occurs during late adolescence or early adulthood

- Is thought to share the same genetic component as anorexia nervosa

- Occurs across all cultures with an abundance of food available

- Other co-morbid medical and psychiatric illnesses can exist

- Estimated prevalence for bulimia nervosa and bulimia-like disorders is 6–8%

The demographics of binge-eating disorder*

- Life-time prevalence of binge-eating disorder is 1–4%

- Occurs in women and men (ratio of 3:2, females:males)

- Binge-eating occurs in approximately one-third of obese men and women

(*can be included as bulimia-like or as obesity; see Chapters 10 and 11.)

 Patient's perspective

'When I was 15, I looked at myself and thought: "I'm too fat, and hate the size of my thighs and bottom." My BMI was then 23. So I started to diet, and got my father to buy an exercise bike, which I rode for an hour each day. In the next year, I exercised a lot but ate normal meals and didn't gain weight. Then I got hepatitis and was in hospital for 6 weeks when I lost weight to a BMI of 20, but it built up to BMI of 21 in a few months—and that's the weight I think I look best at.

So I was happy. I went to university when I was 18 and had a boyfriend. We got on well but I started eating more and exercising less and my weight went up (BMI 23). He said I was getting fat and so did a girl in the class, who was really fat. I don't know if it was what they said, but about then I began to be very aware of women's bodies, and how much they varied in shape. I began to be quite obsessed with body shape and I began to diet. It didn't do much good because my body remained the same shape and I didn't lose any weight although I tried for a year. I think I became convinced that I couldn't eat as much as other people because if I did I would get really fat.

Then my boyfriend and I split up and I was sure it was because I was fat. I tried I don't remember how many diets. I tried staying awake all night because I'd read that mental activity helped lose weight. I even stopped taking vitamin tablets because I thought that there might be calories in the capsules. Nothing worked for me, and my weight stayed between BMI 23 and 25.

I felt the only way that I could really lose weight would be to starve. And I did, but I got so hungry that when I had fasted for 2 or 3 weeks, only drinking fluids, I would binge-out. I used to go out late at night and buy food or if I could, steal it. I tried to induce vomiting after the binge by sticking my fingers down my throat but I couldn't manage it so I started taking laxatives and when, after a binge, my ankles were swollen, I would get diuretic tablets from the doctor. My eating was really out of my control—I really did need help!'

Three years later:

'Looking back, I think that the reason I started binge eating was because of my obsession with dieting, which stemmed from the fact I didn't real-ize in the first place that I wasn't overweight but that I had inherited fatter legs and thighs than the average person.'

Onset of bulimia nervosa

Before the onset of bulimia nervosa, nearly all sufferers, generally when they were between the ages of 14 and 24, have had periods when they restricted their food (intentionally or unintentionally), experimented with 'fad' or 'crazy' diets, or induced vomiting. This in turn led to episodes of binge eating when the woman's control over her food intake weakened. Over time, the frequency and severity of the binge eating increases, as she strives to maintain control over her eating and a bulimia nervosa-like eating disorder develops.

The onset of bulimia nervosa may also be associated with stressful life events that are not related to the woman's concern about body image or weight. An argument, illness, or death in the immediate family, the stress of examinations, a change in job, breakdown of a relationship, divorce, or pregnancy may precipitate the first eating binge. The age of the woman has a bearing on which kind of life events will precipitate binge eating. Family problems are more common precipitants if the woman is a teenager, while above the age of 20, relationship difficulties are more common. Many women who have bulimia nervosa have a normal personality and no detectable psychopathology, but some patients have a personality disorder, which results in the woman having difficulties in her everyday living and coping with the problems her personality causes for her (see page 44). Personality factors may play an important part in the woman's ability to recover and remain free from her illness.

Maintaining bulimia nervosa

Continued attempts to undereat may be one why reason binge eating occurs and may explain why learning 'normal eating' is essential to the management of bulimia nervosa-like disorders. Normally, when a person has eaten the amount of food her body requires, messages from her brain 'turn off' her desire to eat more. As most patients with bulimia diet between eating binges, they are in a 'food-deprived state' and changes in their brain chemistry occur. When a person in a food-deprived state starts eating, the brain messages that normally 'turn off' appetite fail to work so that the person continues eating and overeats, thus commencing an eating binge. This is followed by attempts at further food restriction and a cycle develops (see Chapter 3).

 Fact!

Women who have bulimia nervosa have a low self-esteem.

The psychological dependence on binge eating or vomiting to relieve anxiety, tension, and uncomfortable, dysphoric feelings is discussed later in this chapter (page 165).

Binge eating and panic attacks

Panic attacks are identified by a feeling of agitation and panic that seems to occur for no reason. Some women who suffer from panic attacks and also have bulimia nervosa may use food to cope with the feeling of panic. These women have described that they begin stuffing food into their mouths as soon as the panic attack starts and then vomit quickly. They say that in this way they are able to get over the attack in 2 or 3 minutes.

The eating binge

'It is easy to convince yourself on the day after each binge that that was the last one, and as of today you are never going to binge again. Unfortunately, the nausea and feeling of self-revulsion disappears after a few days, and before you know it, the idea of escape into a session of eating unlimited amounts of anything that takes your fancy gets hold of you again.'

Precipitants of an eating binge

Women report that an eating binge can be precipitated by feelings of:

- tension;
- loneliness;
- unhappiness;
- boredom;
- anxiety;
- a desire to relax;
- the need to escape;
- a craving for food; or
- thinking about or seeing food.

Eating 'bad' food (see Chapter 10) and 'binge' food, which they do not allow themselves to eat at other times, or even eating 'anything' has also been cited by patients as a precipitant to binge eating.

Characteristics of the binge

Most binge eaters are secretive about their behaviour. Many prepare secretively for the binge, or plan for it by hoarding food beforehand. Some women binge only on food available at home, while others buy food especially to eat during episodes of binge eating. Others go out and buy food during a binge session, going from shop to shop and eating as they go. A few will go out late at night to buy food.

In general, the rate at which the woman eats becomes slower as the binge-eating episode proceeds. Initially, most bulimic patients eat their food quickly, some stuffing food frantically into their mouth and often making a considerable mess. Other women are careful to make no mess so that they may avoid detection of their binge eating. The rate of eating during an binge is slower if the woman knows that she will not be disturbed, particularly if she knows she can induce vomiting without being discovered.

The binge may start at any time of the day and end just as suddenly.

Why a binge eating episode ends

The reasons given by women for a binge-eating episode ending include:

* running out of steam;

* fullness;

* discomfort;

* nausea;

* no longer being able to continue to binge secretively;

* having no more food left.

After the binge, most binge eaters promise themselves that they will keep to their strict diet, or will fast and will not repeat the binge. A few fall asleep, but most ('vomiters') take up their usual activities as if the binge had never happened.

Duration and frequency of an eating binge

It is difficult to be certain what bulimia nervosa sufferers mean by the length of a binge-eating episode, but it usually lasts less than 2 hours. Women, especially those who have only recently developed abnormal eating behaviour, perceive their binge eating as occurring in separate episodes; the number of binges on any one day of binge eating ranges from one to six. Some women continue to binge eat at this frequency. Other women, usually those with a long history of binge eating, but having six to 15 episodes a day, each being terminated by vomiting, may describe their episodes as lasting for days or weeks. By this, they mean that the urge to binge eat is continuous and is present even when they go to sleep and on waking, although it is obvious that they do not binge eat continuously.

Food eaten during an eating binge

 Fact!

Binge eaters include food in their binges that they do not allow themselves to eat at other times, i.e. 'bad' food.

The amount, type, and nutritional content of food eaten during a binge vary widely, both within and among individuals.

The amount of food eaten during an eating binge varies considerably, and ranges from three to 30 times the amount of food usually eaten in a day. Many women eat over 10 times the amount of food that they would normally eat each day when not binge eating. This can provide a large amount of energy, exceeding more than 83,700 kJ (20,000 kcal) during days of 'bad binge eating'. Those who eat large quantities of food are more likely to reach higher body weights, irrespective of the amount of vomiting.

Many binge eaters claim they go on eating until they have eaten all of the food available. However, when this claim is analysed, it is found that they are usually referring only to what they describe as 'binge' or 'bad' foods. Only a few actually eat everything in the cupboards and fridge.

Contrary to most binge eaters' impressions that the food eaten during binges is exceptionally high in fat, analysis of records of food actually consumed in a binge has revealed that they are just as likely to contain excessive amounts of carbohydrate or protein. The amount, type, and nutritional content of the food eaten during a binge may be entirely dependent on what is available in the home (see example in the box below), or partly for ease of vomiting. Some women will eat anything that is available, including tinned food, baby food, frozen food, and scraps from rubbish bins.

Example of food eaten during a 'bad day' of binge eating over a period of 8 hours

3 loaves bread, 6 large potatoes (chips), 1 jar honey, 1 jar anchovies (on bread), 1 pkt rolled oats, large pancake mix, 1 pkt macaroni, 2 instant puddings, 1 bag nuts, 1 large pkt Rice Bubbles, 1 tub margarine, oil (for cooking), 2 cartons milk (in porridge, in drink), 2 large containers ice-cream, 8 sausages, 4 onions, 12 eggs (in milkshake, scrambled eggs), large pkt

liquorice allsorts, 2 family-size blocks chocolate, 1 pkt dried figs, 2 pkts sweets, 6 'health bars', assorted cream cakes (up to 12) eaten while shopping, sultanas (on bread or in porridge), leftovers found in fridge, 1 bottle orange cordial.

This amount of food gives a total of:

- Energy: 226,070 kJ (54,000 kcal)

- Protein: 1071 g

- Fat: 1964 g

- Carbohydrate: 14,834 g

How do binge eaters try to resist binge eating?

Nearly every binge eater has attempted, at times, to resist the urge to binge. The methods chosen to resist the urge to binge eat vary considerably. Some women feel a reduced urge if they:

- keep no food in the house;

- avoid food shops;

- have no money to spend;

- avoid cooking or going into the kitchen;

- study where no food is available (e.g. library);

- plan to be occupied at all times;

- knit;

- become absorbed with the Internet or computer games;

- have a jigsaw puzzle or sudoko to do;

- telephone friends;

- go out and meet people;

- do not drink excess alcohol;

- do not sit down to watch television when they get home late;

- do not eat in front of television;

- always go straight to the bedroom if they get home late;

- have a shower or bath or wash their hair;

- go for a walk;

- exercise;

- plan to be occupied during 'at risk' times;

- work longer hours in a job where no food is available;

- follow a normal menu plan.

A few women will use exercise as a way of avoiding binge eating (see *Patient's perspective*: Ellen). They may spend long hours at the gym or run many miles every day.

 Patient's perspective

Ellen exercised to avoid binge eating. She wrote:

'The running was a great help to me in overcoming my eating problems and increasing self-esteem. I reached the point where going fast was more important than looking good, and of course an athlete has to eat well to race well. Also, I think the ability to be aggressive in training and racing and to push my body to its limits provided an outlet for the tension and anxiety that I used to release as bulimia.

I must admit to the occasional bulimic episode, perhaps once or twice a year. There are other times when I feel like it, but don't have the time or opportunity. These times are usually when I am angry but unable to express it; or feel out of control of my life or my time; or feel anxious or depressed. I think anger usually has something to do with it—again, I guess running was a good outlet for aggression, since when I was racing regularly the thought never entered my mind. I still do not cope very well with putting on weight. I gained about 3 kg during the first year (due to relative inactivity), but lost it quickly after the exams (lots of sport). I felt quite uncomfortable, physically and psychologically, at that weight. I wish it didn't matter to me, but it still does. However, I don't feel out of control, because I know that I can lose it easily.'

Strategies used by bulimia nervosa sufferers to control weight

Women who binge eat are aware that obesity is inevitable if they continue their behaviour and do not take measures to control their weight. For patients with bulimia nervosa, their fear of fatness is as great as their love of food. Faced with this dilemma, two strategies are available to them. The first is to reduce the amount of energy absorbed from the food they eat by inducing vomiting during and after binge eating, and between binges. The second method is to diet strictly and exercise between binges. The prolonged, regular use of laxatives to control weight gain among patients with bulimia nervosa is declining in popularity, as women are learning how ineffective they are in controlling body weight (see Table 9.1). The quantity of laxatives taken varies from double the recommended dose, taken immediately after an eating binge, to 'handfuls' of tablets every day. Using diuretic 'fluid' tablets to feel less bloated and uncomfortable is seldom seen nowadays.

Table 9.1. Potentially dangerous methods of compensating for binge eating among 26 patients with anorexia nervosa and 106 who were bulimia nervosa-like over the previous 3 months

	Women binge eating (more than twice a week) (%)	
	BMI less than 17.5 kg/m^2 (*n*=26)	BMI more than 17.5 kg/m^2 (*n*=106)
Self-induced vomiting:		
never	15	28
less than twice a week	8	6
more than twice a week	77	66
(daily)	(39)	(51)
Laxatives:		
never	69	72
less than twice a week	23	21
more than twice a week	8	7
(daily)	(0)	(11)
Alcohol:		
binge drink	15	30
used for shape/weight	0	2
Recreational drugs:		
used	8	15
used for shape/weight	8	6

About 60% of binge eaters briefly try commercial 'slimming pills', which often contain some form of laxative, and a few take appetite-suppressing medications (stimulants), which have an addictive property. The use of 'party' drugs such as 'ecstasy' or 'ice' for weight control is increasing.

Some binge eaters will try to avoid eating binges by using alcohol (see *Patient's perspective*: Penny) or other drugs. A few women who develop a drug or alcohol dependence may recover from their eating disorder, but the drug or alcohol problem may persist for years and may require treatment.

 Patient's perspective

Penny described her story as follows:

'I really started binge eating when I was about 12. Before that I had bought lots of sweets, candies, and lollies, because Mum gave me a lot of pocket money—but all kids do that. Then, when I was about 12, I started dieting and began binge eating. I remember that I used to eat my packed lunch on the way to school and then scrounge food from the other kids. By the time I was 14, I was a real binge eater. After a binge I would vomit, and after a time I could vomit without putting my fingers down my throat. I still can, but I don't do it. What with study and fixing up binge eating, I didn't have time for friends. But it didn't seem to matter, I just had to binge eat and I did, and then I vomited so that I wouldn't put on weight.

That went on until I was 20. I had this job—it was so boring and I hated it. One day after an eating binge, I was so agitated I drank half a bottle of wine. It worked wonders. It steadied my nerves and I felt better. I started thinking that if I had a drink I wouldn't need to binge eat. I bought a bottle of whisky and kept it in my wardrobe. When thoughts of food and putting on weight became overwhelming, I'd drink some alcohol and they would be less insistent. That's how I stopped binge eating. I went on vomiting—it's easy to do when you know how and my weight dropped from a BMI of 26 to a BMI of 18. When I was drinking, I was much more relaxed and began to go out with friends.

About this time I realized I was wasting my life so I left the dull job and stopped drinking, except on social occasions when I would binge drink, or eat all the food I could. I guess the occasions gave me permission to indulge my needs. I started a course, which was hard work, and one day I began binge eating again. It was just after my 21st birthday when I had got drunk and had horrified my parents. Soon I was binge eating three or more times a week. I started vomiting again and took large doses of laxatives. Because I was scared that I would put on weight even after what I was doing, I began to jog and was soon running 10 km a day. It seemed to help. When I was jogging I stopped thinking about food and my weight, which stayed at a BMI of 21. Because of the vomiting, my teeth were going bad, but I couldn't stop vomiting after an eating binge; it made me feel relaxed. And if I was having problems, or was worried, I'd drop into the pub and have a few quick drinks. Mind you, I was worried that I might be an alcoholic.

The next year I met Wayne and we moved in together. It was great at first but I still needed to binge, and I did, often every day, and I kept a bottle or two of whisky hidden at home, just in case I needed a drink. When Wayne found out he was furious and I felt it was time I saw a doctor.'

Over the next 3 years, Penny remained in outpatient treatment, she occasionally binge ate and returned twice briefly to her previous behaviour of binge eating three or more times a week and using alcohol. Her weight remained stable at around a BMI of 21, and she led an active social life. She was eventually head-hunted for a very good executive position in another firm.

Self-induced vomiting

'I find it easy to pinpoint the beginning of my illness. It began with an experience concerning one of my 15th birthday presents: a box of chocolates. I was at an age where pressures for social acceptance were, to me, immense, and pencil thinness, to me, was a prerequisite for social acceptance and self-confidence. I ate some of my birthday chocolates and was offered a suggestion by my mother: "If you don't want to get fat, stick your fingers down your throat." Maybe this statement has more relevance than I'd previously thought. Mum's simple statement triggered off every emotional fear within me: "I'll be fat—socially unacceptable—ugly—have no self-confidence—no self-esteem . . .".'

Food eaten during a binge is sometimes selected because it is easy to 'stuff down' at the beginning of a binge and easy to vomit up. Some of our binge eaters said that their binges consisted mainly of soft, milky, or fluid foods, whereas others said they used such foods merely as a means to assist vomiting, and ate them towards the end of the binge. Some of the reasons given by patients for inducing vomiting are given in Table 9.2.

Initially vomiting is achieved by stuffing the fingers or a spoon into the throat, but later many women can induce vomiting by inducing a strong contraction of the diaphragm and abdominal muscles to force the contents of the stomach into the oesophagus and then to vomit. In each episode of vomiting, many women regurgitate between one and ten times until they are certain that all of the food has been brought up. Some women use 'markers', beginning a binge with food such as red apple skin, lettuce, or liquorice that they can recognize in the vomit. A number of patients also use 'wash-out techniques', where they keep drinking water and regurgitating until there is no residue of food in their stomach, a process that can last up to half an hour. In most cases, the vomiting episodes last from 5 to 30 minutes, depending on ease of vomiting and quantity of food eaten.

Table 9.2 Reasons given by anorexia nervosa-like and bulimia nervosa-like patients for inducing vomiting

Reason for inducing vomiting	Important (%)	Very important (%)
To get rid of food eaten	4.2	91.7
To prevent weight gain	0.0	87.5
To feel in control	8.3	79.2
To lose weight	4.2	66.7
To relieve anxious/agitated feelings	12.5	62.5
To release stress	16.7	58.3
To feel empty inside	20.8	54.2
To relieve depressed feelings	20.8	50.0
To stop anger	16.7	50.0
To feel better mentally	25.0	45.8
To feel good	20.8	41.7
To help concentration	12.5	20.8
To stop panic attacks	8.3	20.8

Fact!

Vomiting is not 100% efficient at stopping food being absorbed.

In spite of these methods to ensure that vomiting is efficient, it does not completely prevent the absorption of foods, particularly the simple sugars that are absorbed quite quickly.

The physical effects of self-induced vomiting

Women who habitually binge eat and induce vomiting may develop a variety of symptoms that can be seen or experienced (see box below).

Physical and psychological changes that may accompany bulimia nervosa

- Fatigue, irritability, anger

- Lethargy

- Nausea and headache

- Abdominal discomfort and bloating

- Constipation, irritable bowel

- Swelling of hands and feet

- Menstrual irregularity

- Dry skin

- Dehydration

- Calluses on the back of fingers (from inducing vomiting)

- Swollen salivary (parotid) glands (puffy face)

- Inflammation of the stomach and oesophagus

- Dyspepsia

- Gastro-oesophageal (acid) reflux

- Blood in vomit

- Dental enamel erosion leading to chipped, 'moth-eaten' teeth (see *Patient's perspective*: Charlie)

- Electrolyte disturbance, cardiac arrhythmias, renal problems (see page 111)

 Patient's perspective

Charlie recovered from bulimia nervosa. Her father wrote to thank us for the efforts we had made to help her recover.

'The cost of inpatient treatment was high,' he wrote, 'but I do not begrudge that. What I do begrudge is what I had to pay to the dentist to repair the damage Charlie had done to her teeth. Before she became ill, she had the most beautiful teeth. They will never be the same, even with the dental care they have received'.

 Fact!

Initial weight gain after stopping vomiting is all fluid (due to rehydration).

When a woman stops vomiting she may suffer abdominal cramps, bloating, constipation or diarrhoea, and may feel exhausted or become very agitated. These 'withdrawal' symptoms cease after 10 days. Three weeks later, she is no longer agitated or fatigued, and usually says that she feels better than she has done for years.

Abuse of laxatives, slimming tablets, and diuretics

All that laxatives do is cause the body to lose fluid, not energy. This is followed by rebound water retention so that the person's body weight may be higher after taking laxatives than it was before.

Stopping laxative abuse is also followed by 'withdrawal' symptoms, which are similar to those that follow the cessation of self-induced vomiting. These are constipation, abdominal cramps, abdominal bloating, agitation, and feeling 'awful'. A woman needs to be reassured that these symptoms, which usually occur, are normal and will usually cease after 10 days.

Diuretics rid the body of water and electrolytes. The relief they provide from feeling 'full' is temporary and their regular use may lead to short-term or long-term persistent fluid retention when they are discontinued.

Menstrual disturbances

Many binge eaters develop menstrual irregularities, although, in contrast to women who have anorexia nervosa, their body weight is usually in the normal range for age and height, or they are overweight. About 40% of women who have bulimia nervosa develop irregular menstruation and in another 20%, menstruation ceases. These women need reassurance that menstruation will become normal when their body weight stabilizes and when they have ceased to use dangerous methods of weight control, including intermittent starvation and excessive exercise (see Chapter 7). Doctors may also suggest testing for polycystic ovarian syndrome in a few women.

Psychological effects of binge eating

'I became increasingly aware of my increasing ability to relieve life's pressure through the intake of food. Although the induction of vomiting continued to be traumatic, the relief, and the euphoria afterwards, were, to me, of no comparison to it.'

Before starting to binge eat, most women feel tense and anxious, have palpitations, or begin sweating. During the binge, most binge eaters feel a sense of freedom; the anxiety, worry, or unpleasant feeling they had been experiencing lifts and they no longer have anxious or negative thoughts. Women can describe this as relief, escape, 'time out', or numbness. If the woman chooses to induce vomiting, she may also reduce tension and dysphoria with the act of vomiting (Table 9.2). At the end of the binge, most binge eaters feel less tense and anxious, but may not like themselves because of what they have done to their bodies. They may feel guilty about inducing vomiting and may panic that the binge may induce a weight gain. This in turn may lead to further anxiety and

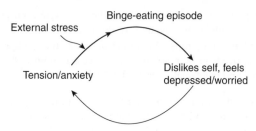

Figure 9.1 The psychological circle of binge eating

tension, with the result that they may start binge eating once again. A vicious circle is established (Figure 9.1).

If a binge eater is unable to relieve her anxiety and tension, for example, if the person is interrupted or discovered when binge eating, her behaviour may change to agitation, anger, or aggression.

It is also apparent that if a woman with bulimia nervosa does not recognize the tension and anxiety, or has no other ways of coping with them, she easily enters a vicious circle and becomes a frequent binge eater. As will be seen, a major objective of treatment is to break this self-perpetuating circle of eating behaviour.

Effect of bulimia nervosa on body weight

Before developing the eating disorder, the body weight of most binge eaters is within the normal range. About 20% are overweight or obese, and a similar proportion is underweight, often being diagnosed as having anorexia nervosa. After starting binge eating, many of the women show frequent swings in body weight.

 Fact!

Binge eating occurs among obese women and women of normal body weight, and some patients with anorexia nervosa binge eat.

Patient's perspective

Jane started dieting at the age of 16 to control her weight. At first, she had a small, steady loss in weight. At the age of 17, she began binge eating and for the next 6 years she alternated between binge eating and strict, almost starvation diets, with resulting large swings in weight of up to 19 kg (42 lb or 3 st). When her weight was below 55 kg (121 lb or 8 st 9 lb), her menstrual periods ceased, but they returned when her weight exceeded that value. On two occasions of about 2 weeks' duration, her weight fell to a BMI of 15, placing her into the clinically defined category of anorexia nervosa.

Other binge eaters control their weight fluctuations to within 3 kg (6½ lb) by dieting and exercising excessively between binges, or by using vomiting and purging to try to prevent absorption of the food eaten during a binge. Women who induce vomiting and binge eat large amounts of food are usually overweight, while the weight of women whose binges are small is usually in the normal range, irrespective of how efficient they are at inducing vomiting.

Sexuality

'Often I used to go out and eat for my sensual sexual experience of the day. I actually would be turned on by it.'

It appears that many women who have an eating disorder perceive an association between eating and sexuality. The sexual knowledge, attitudes, and behaviour of women with binge-eating disorders are very varied. Their sexual activity can:

- mirror their eating-disordered behaviour: increased sexual activity is associated with increased vomiting and binge eating; or

- the eating disorder can replace sexual behaviour: when they are binge eating, they are not interested in sexual activity.

If a woman is not menstruating, her libido will be low and she may experience a lack of vaginal lubrication (see page 124).

Women who have been abused may need additional help to overcome sexual and relationship problems. They may avoid relationships and sexual matters (like patients with anorexia nervosa), or they may take risks and become sexually promiscuous.

Marriage and children

For the woman who marries when she has active bulimia nervosa, the chance that the marriage will break down is double that of other women, although this is not the case if she marries before she develops bulimia nervosa, or after recovery. For conception, pregnancy, and the postnatal period in bulimic women, see Chapter 4. Prenatal and postnatal distress is more common if the woman has a current eating disorder.

10

Treatment and outcome of bulimia and bulimia nervosa-like disorders

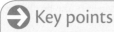 Key points

- Ten to 15 years after treatment for bulimia nervosa, 80% of patients are improved or recovered; relapses are common, especially in the first 2 years

- Treatment involves nutritional counselling, learning 'normal' structured eating, and ceasing weight-losing behaviour; monitoring of mood and behaviour is important

- Treatment involves supportive psychotherapy with cognitive behaviour therapy (CBT)

- Additional psychological therapies and techniques help the woman manage her moods and behaviour while fulfilling the aims of treatment

- Ongoing psychological treatment helps her learn to cope with stress, anxiety, and dysphoric moods without using food and eating-disordered behaviours

- Most patients with bulimia nervosa and with bulimia nervosa-like disorders are treated as outpatients

- Exercise should be monitored throughout the treatment

'Normality is the heaven for which I strive. Perhaps I will have it some day. I certainly haven't given up. This, however, is not as simple as it sounds to a binge eater. It should be so easy to forget about counting calories and just eat three normal meals every day, but somehow the reassurance of knowing that you didn't eat more than your allowed calories is necessary. Without this reassurance, confusion can result, bringing on a binge. Counting calories doesn't mean dieting or denying yourself fattening foods—it simply means controlling your overall food intake and allowing for these fattening extras in your diet. It can stop the guilt associated with eating high-calorie items, a guilt which may be the cause of a binge.'

Aims of treatment

The aims of the treatment of bulimia nervosa are described in the box below.

- ◆ To help the woman acquire new attitudes to food, eating, body shape, and weight

- ◆ To help her reduce her preoccupation with food

- ◆ To persuade her to eat a meal three times a day, with two or three snacks

- ◆ To understand the benefits of eating at regular times

- ◆ To help her avoid inappropriate methods for losing weight such as self-induced vomiting, laxative abuse, and compulsive exercise

- ◆ To help her obtain insight into her mood changes and to learn to cope with these moods using ways other than binge eating

- ◆ To help her recognize what precipitates her binge eating

- ◆ To help her find ways to cope with her problems, feelings, and moods, other than resorting to binge eating, vomiting, or excess exercise

- ◆ To help her improve her self-esteem

- ◆ To provide support and reassurance

The one major element required for recovery from bulimia is a desperate will to live normally. The aims of treatment suggest that the binge eater needs to:

- be motivated to recover;

- learn that dieting is unnecessary;

- learn that most foods can be eaten in moderate quantities without a dramatic change in weight;

- eat at least three meals a day;

- stop dividing foods into 'good' and 'bad' foods;

- discontinue vomiting and weight-losing behaviour;

- understand that urges to binge eat certain foods may persist for many months;

- meet with the therapist each week, or every 2 weeks, to plan for the next period;

- learn to like herself; and

- be accepting and cope with her feelings, even distressing feelings.

Cognitive behavioural therapy

The most successful psychological treatment to date for bulimia nervosa is the cognitive behavioural therapy (CBT) model in association with supportive psychotherapy. The model is continually being modified as new psychological techniques are introduced. CBT is described on page 97. Before starting treatment, the history of the eating disorder and the woman's physical condition is checked so that any specific needs can be addressed during CBT treatment. Some of these needs will be discussed in this chapter. During the interview, the therapist (or the dietician) stresses the importance of keeping a mood diary and a food diary in the first weeks of treatment (see page 96).

 Fact!

Keeping a daily mood, food, and behaviour diary is a necessary part of treatment.

The therapist discusses the mood diary with the patient and helps her separate her mood and how she feels from food; in other words, the therapist helps her discover that her moods and feelings are not dependent on whether she will eat, what she has eaten, whether she has dieted, or whether she feels 'fat' and unattractive.

The dietician discusses the food diary with the woman and encourages her to stop weighing herself more than once a week, counting units of energy, reading food labels, cooking for others, and indulging in behaviours that keep her thinking about food and weight. The basic aspects of CBT are outlined in the box below. In practice, stage I and stage II of CBT overlap. When a woman is completing her daily diaries and discussing these with her therapist, she gains insight into her behaviour and realizes that some of her beliefs and fears are no longer valid. This allows her to challenge her beliefs and change her behaviour.

A summary of CBT

Preliminary

The therapist:

1. Takes a comprehensive history of the eating disorder, checks the patient's physical, reproductive, and psychological health, her family history, and explores her attitudes to her eating problem.

2. Establishes trust between the patient and herself, and introduces her to a dietician.

Stage I: weeks 1–6 (meetings once or twice each week)

The therapist:

1. Persuades the patient to record in detail everything she eats, at what times she eats and how much, and what thoughts and feelings she has during eating. (Food and mood diaries (see Table 6.3) may be chosen or one of the other records shown in the self-help manuals.) The recorded information is discussed at the weekly meetings.

2. Offers alternative behavioural choices to help the patient resist binge eating.

The therapist asks the patient to meet with the dietician, who:

1. Persuades her to eat food at regular intervals and not to binge eat.

2. Teaches her about food and eating behaviour.

Stage II: weeks 6–12

The therapist:

1. Helps the patient explore why she started binge eating.

2. Helps her change her thoughts about problems with her eating behaviour, her shape, and her weight.

3. Helps her develop skills to deal with difficulties that trigger binges.

4. Discusses with the patient the role (if any) of her family, partner, and social situation.

The dietician:

1. Starts gradually introducing avoided foods (which the patient perceives as 'bad') into her diet.

2. Gradually eliminates all forms of strict dieting.

Stage III: weeks 12–24

At this stage most patients have not fully recovered. The therapist reassures the patient that progress will continue and reassures her that, even when the programme finishes, help will be readily available if her symptoms return or worsen, or if she has any further problems.

With thanks to Christopher Fairburn for permission to paraphrase his summary of CBT, which he has developed and tested since 1980.

Combined psychological therapies

Other psychological therapeutic techniques are also introduced into the CBT model. The eclectic approach is to assess each woman individually and evaluate the possible usefulness of the various therapies for the woman: nutritional therapy, antidepressant medication (selective serotonin reuptake inhibitors or SSRIs), behavioural therapy, interpersonal therapy, motivational therapy, anxiety management, life skills, exercise, family or marital therapies, and the newer psychological techniques of mindfulness, acceptance and commitment, and schema therapy (see pages 97–9). Any combination of these can be employed at the same time or at different stages of treatment. As new psychological techniques are introduced, their possible usefulness can be assessed and introduced for individual patients. In clinical practice, a combination of approaches is used, particularly if treatment is provided by a team of people trained in different disciplines. Studies of treatment involving a combination of therapies are showing promising results.

Fact!

Dialectical behaviour therapy is useful for bulimic women with impulsive personality difficulties.

Carer support

Support groups for parents, siblings, and partners are also important, particularly soon after the problem has been discovered or while the woman is being treated in hospital. It is reassuring for parents and partners to know that other people have a daughter, sister, or partner with similar problems, and to be able to share and talk through their fears and hopes. They also need to feel that they can have contact and communicate with the people who are helping their daughter or partner. It is hard for most people to understand why sufferers cannot just 'change their behaviour' and 'get better'.

Continuing supportive psychotherapy

The importance of continuing support from the therapist cannot be overemphasized, as relapses in the first 2 years of treatment may occur. Changes to the flexible structured eating patterns that a woman has learnt to unstructured eating should be discouraged. For this reason, she should also avoid long holidays or trips overseas. In an unfamiliar environment, with the loss of routine, frequent new experiences, and different foods, it is common for bulimic patients to feel that they have lost control of their body weight and to revert to a pattern of binge eating, self-induced vomiting, and purgation. Because of the fear of returning to binge eating, some women recovering from bulimia nervosa respond by not eating and then become ill, with extreme weight loss, and need to return home quickly (see *Patient's perspective*: Kara in Chapter 8).

During psychotherapy, emphasis is placed on allowing the woman to learn to cope with problems and crises that may occur without relapsing into old patterns of behaviour. She is encouraged to express her feelings and to talk about emotional material. This may involve current interactions with her family, partner, or friends, as well as with past unpleasant events such as being bullied at school, feeling abandoned by a parent as a child, or experiencing physical or sexual abuse. The therapist must have the skills to work with a range of problems once they have been raised.

During the time that a woman is suffering from bulimia nervosa, she should talk to her therapist if she is considering taking a job that is associated with food, such as waitressing, because preparing or serving food is likely to provoke an episode of binge eating. Similarly, jobs associated with exercise and body shape, such as becoming an exercise instructor or personal trainer, may be too much of a challenge for the woman at that time.

Changing attitudes to food, shape, and weight

'In the back of my mind, I still feel that—should events one day go bad in my life—I could return to the binge eating as before. If there was too much pressure, worries, or if I couldn't cope with problems, food is the crutch to keep me going. It would have to be very bad, but I also think I would seek help from my counsellors to keep me from turning entirely to food. I'm not sure—it exists as a possibility. Certainly, if I was bored, unhappy with my lifestyle (for example, stuck in a little house with a baby and no friends or money to buy things), or doing things I did not really want to do, food or eating might become the only interesting facet of life (as they were once to me). But I hope not. And I think—I really think—I'll make it without food in the long run.'

'Good' and 'bad' foods

Some patients need help to learn to incorporate social eating back into their lifestyle. The fewer diet restrictions there are, the easier this is. It also means giving up the distinction between 'good' and 'bad' foods. Bad foods are perceived by patients with bulimia nervosa to be foods that contain fat or are high in carbohydrates. Some examples of foods that our patients described as good and bad are listed in Table 10.1. This table shows that many of the 'good' foods are those recommended by expert committees concerned with preventing obesity, heart disease, and diabetes. However, many patients with eating disorders have ideas about foods that are not accurate and the likelihood of a woman being able to resist eating all of the foods on the 'bad' list over a long period of time is very low. Learning to eat all foods in moderation at meal times or on social occasions, rather than only during binge eating, is an important action for women who are recovering from bulimia nervosa to learn.

Table 10.1 The perception of 'good' and 'bad' foods by women who have eating disorders

'Bad' foods	'Good' foods
Energy-dense foods	High-fibre foods
Foods containing fat	Foods with no fat content
Take-away ('junk') foods	Vegetables, but not potatoes
Snack foods	Fruit
Dairy products, including milk and cheese	Yoghurt
Red meat	Chicken and fish
Bread and biscuits, cakes	Diet biscuits
Sweets, lollies, candies, and chocolate Ice-cream	Anything bought in a health food shop, including honey

Normal and abnormal eating

The main treatment objectives are to help the bulimia nervosa sufferer change her thoughts about food, her body shape, and her weight, and to persuade her to eat normally. Many bulimic women have forgotten what normal eating is and need encouragement and help to change their thoughts about normal and abnormal eating. The following box describes what normal eating involves and may help them to achieve this objective.

Normal eating behaviour

Normal eating **is**:

- eating at least three meals a day, with two or three snacks;

- eating a wide variety of foods as part of a balanced and flexible diet;

- eating more of the foods whose taste and texture you enjoy when you wish to;

- eating more than you feel the need to eat on some occasions (overeating);

- eating less than you need on some occasions (undereating);

- eating in a flexible way so that it does not interfere with your work, study, or social life, and vice versa;

- eating or not eating on occasions when you feel unhappy, 'bad', or tense;

- eating, when out socially, in a similar manner to the other people in the group;

- eating at fast food outlets occasionally when you wish to or are with friends;

- being aware that eating is not the most important thing in life, but that it is important for good health, and physical and mental well-being;

- being able to prepare food for yourself and others without feeling anxious;

- knowing what portions of food and size of meals are appropriate in different circumstances.

Normal eating **is not**:

- dieting;

- counting calories (kilojoules), weighing food, or following a strict diet (unless medically indicated);

- reading food labels;

- eating to lose weight, but eating to remain in a stable weight range appropriate for your body; if you are obese, you will lose weight if you eat 'normally';

- aiming to eat a diet containing no fat;

- eating low-energy substitute foods, e.g. diet biscuits rather than bread;

- feeling when you eat a particular food that you will be unable to stop until it is all eaten;

- having to weigh yourself for reassurance;

- avoiding eating because you do not know what the food contains;

- playing 'games' with yourself to prevent eating certain foods, e.g. saying 'dairy products make me feel nauseous';

- being obsessed with food.

 Patient's perspective

Maggie described her eating behaviour as follows:

'The beauty of bulimia always seemed to be that I could eat as much as I wanted, because I knew I could get rid of it either through vomiting, exercise, laxatives, or starving. For the last 6 years, I have used food as my comfort whenever I felt angry, sad, anxious, bored, or felt any uneasy feeling. I knew food would make me feel better instantly. I would eat my favourite foods. I would buy them especially for a binge. Chocolates, Twisties, chips, cakes, lollies, pies, sausage rolls, cheese dips, and biscuits—all foods that I class in the "bad food" category. I would eat until I felt better, but then I would start to feel bad again and my behaviours, like vomiting, would erase those bad feelings almost instantly.

I would say at the end of every binge: "This is the last time I will ever do this," and I would go for days when I wouldn't eat anything. I would just drink water. Then I would eat things that I classed as "good" foods—fruit, diet foods, vegetables, foods with the least amounts of calories and fat. Or maybe for a week I would just eat a chocolate bar every day.

But then I would build back up to a binge again. All the bad food would come back out again. Control was lost in every way. And I thought this was normal eating.'

 Fact!

Structured eating is eating appropriate amounts at meal and snack times that are not too far apart.

Unstructured eating is eating at any time and 'grazing'.

Avoiding weight-losing behaviour

Unintentional undereating

Women who binge eat do not know how much food they need to eat when they are no longer binge eating. They are surprised at the amount of food required and convinced that this amount will cause weight gain. Learning they have been aiming to undereat allows them to challenge their old patterns of eating. It also helps them understand that hunger can be a precipitant to binge eating, even for women who do not use extreme methods of weight control. Binge eaters are usually intentionally or unintentionally undereating between binge-eating episodes.

Intentional weight-losing behaviours

Structured, normal eating is needed when stopping weight-losing behaviours. Many women who binge eat are willing, at least initially, to try to change their behaviour, and are reassured when they learn about the effects that may occur. Most are unaware that they may gain 'weight' when they cease the behaviour, as a result of retaining fluid in their body. Seeing this apparent weight gain causes the woman to panic and to try and gain control by returning to her weight-losing behaviour.

Women find it helpful to know the 'withdrawal' symptoms after stopping their weight-losing behaviour. The symptoms that may occur following cessation of strict dieting, starvation, excessive exercise, vomiting, and laxative use are:

◆ bloating;

◆ abdominal fullness;

◆ abdominal discomfort, pain, and cramps;

◆ nausea;

◆ constipation;

◆ an irritable bowel;

◆ dyspepsia (indigestion);

◆ regurgitation;

◆ 'feeling fat';

* fatigue;

* agitation.

Suggestion: Do not weigh yourself when you are trying to stop weight-losing behaviour.

Suggestion: A hot pack on the abdomen can help reduce the symptoms after meals.

After 10 days of avoiding the behaviours mentioned, most patients usually feel comfortable, and after 3 weeks they usually report feeling better than they ever have and they feel energetic. It can take patients time to find the confidence to stop their behaviour completely, because they fear a rapid weight increase and loss of control of their eating. It is difficult for them to believe that their binge eating will lessen if they are eating normally and their weight-losing behaviour stops. Inpatient treatment may be needed for some women to achieve this objective.

Self-induced vomiting

Some women, particularly those with a long history of bulimia nervosa, will explain that they 'binge' only so that they can induce vomiting. They become 'addicted' to vomiting to reduce anxiety and tension. They allow themselves to stop binge eating, but they maintain their vomiting as a quick and effective method of coping with these unpleasant feelings. Acceptance of these feelings and learning to stay with them is part of treatment (see also panic attacks on page 153).

Dysphoric moods

Recognition of negative (dysphoric) moods

Patients describe anxiety, tension, and uncomfortable moods prior to binge eating. In most patients, the negative mood is relieved during the binge or after vomiting (see pages 165–6). Recognition by the patient of the association between unpleasant moods and relief from them by binge eating assists her to find other, more appropriate ways of coping with tension. Therapies aimed at teaching relaxation can help people to recognize their anxiety and stress. Many patients find relaxation difficult at any time and almost impossible prior to a binge when they are most agitated and tense. The practice of acceptance and commitment, and mindfulness techniques, are useful in recovery.

As the frequency of binge eating decreases, and the woman has more understanding of the connection between moods and eating, she can reorganize her lifestyle to minimize eating due to tension or stress; for example, when examinations are approaching, she can do this by working more consistently without a last-minute cram and by studying in a place that does not have easy access to food. Eating is good for procrastination; it does not eliminate the cause of the anxiety.

Antidepressant drugs and bulimia nervosa

Evidence from trials suggests that antidepressants are of limited benefit in the treatment of bulimia nervosa. The antidepressant drugs that increase brain serotonin (SSRIs) do help a small number of women with bulimia nervosa to reduce binge eating in the short term. Interestingly, the women who do respond are no more likely to be suffering from symptoms of depression than the women who do not respond favourably. The theory linking serotonin to binge eating is discussed in Chapter 3 (page 45). Patients should discuss medication with their therapist.

 Patient's perspective

'I still have binges now—but they are shorter, they cause me less remorse and guilt, and I consume less food during them than before. I am fuller sooner. They also relieve my anxious feelings better. I have the binge and I feel relieved. I can even sit and watch television for the rest of the night without continuing to eat, because I am satisfied.

When I was caught up in it before, the night would dissolve into an endless foray in and out of the kitchen. I might stop for 1–2 hours (when absolutely full) but restart eating later. Now, I usually stop and that's it—no more.

If I want to, I can stop the binge before it starts, or even at a point during it. But I have to say to myself: "Why are you doing this?" "What's the matter?" "What are you trying to say to yourself?" or "What are you unhappy about?"

Often the answer comes easily—"I'm unhappy about Bill, I miss him," or "I'm hassled. There are too many things to do and I don't know if I can do them all in time," or "My mother-in-law was here today and she annoys me. She seems to take over our house (even though I know she doesn't) and when she's here everything revolves around her" (she's a semi-invalid).

Sometimes I don't know why I'm binge eating (unlike before when I *never* knew why I was binge eating). And then I can't stop the binge.

Now the binges don't affect my weight that much. Firstly, they mean less food intake. Secondly, I can make up by eating sparingly the next day (and I usually am not hungry for a while). Thirdly, I can run or play tennis to adjust my weight and enjoy the exercise.

How strange to feel "satisfied" and happy with your life! It is the most superb feeling, to feel good about yourself!

I am pleased with my body and what it can do for me (in terms of sport or sex). I have treated myself to the luxury of new, fashionable, trendy clothes—a joy from the days when I wore discreet plain clothes because a fat person had no right to be sexual. I know my body attracts men. I can feel the "vibrations" or I can feel them watching me sometimes. This confirms my feelings of self-confidence in myself but also perhaps suggests that the new-found sexuality is showing. I feel a "complete" person—all the pieces are there fitting together correctly—including the sexual part of me—and I guess it shows.

Binges for me are also a way to relax. I always keep little activities to do around the house so I am "busy" and occupied away from food. But if I am tired or don't want to do them, then sometimes I'm stuck. I want to unwind and food is a good way. It involves little mental effort, it calms the nervous feeling in my stomach, and it takes my mind away from work or troubles.'

Recognition of precipitants

Suggestion: Record the current things that start a binge.

The patient and the therapist explore and discuss those factors, such as marital and family stress (see page 154), loneliness, tenseness, and boredom, that have precipitated binge eating in the past and may still do so. Recognition of precipitants of binge eating helps patients to reorganize their lifestyle either to avoid these situations, to put up with their feelings, or to find other ways of coping at these times. It is interesting that as patients improve they recognize hunger as a precipitant but they also explain that previously they had trouble recognizing accurate cues for hunger and satiation (see *Patient's perspective*: Yvonne on page 191).

Encouragement of resistance behaviour

Suggestion: List the ways you can use to resist binge eating.

Most binge eaters have tried ways of resisting binge eating (see page 157). Some of the less-extreme behaviours can be used successfully at times by different patients, and can be included in treatment programmes. Patients may find that more structure and planning in their day-to-day living is helpful, e.g. meeting a friend on the way home from work. Sensible exercise can be promoted for most sufferers, but the exercise needs to be controlled, as some patients are at risk of developing an exercise disorder (see page 31), which may replace, or coexist with, the eating disorder. The chosen exercise regimen must be perceived by the woman as enjoyable and should preferably involve other people rather than being a solitary activity. Taking up new interests also helps patients to feel better about themselves and to feel more like other people.

Treatment of the physical symptoms

Dehydration and electrolyte disturbance

Most bulimia patients require little medical treatment for their physical symptoms. When treatment is needed, it is usually because the woman is dehydrated, has an electrolyte disturbance or has a vitamin deficiency because of 'starvation diets', self-induced vomiting, or abuse of laxatives. This is explained in Chapter 7 (pages 111–12). In a few cases, treatment is needed because of a suicide attempt or self-harm.

Management of gynaecological problems

Many women with bulimia nervosa have disordered menstruation. Their menstrual periods either cease or occur only infrequently. Investigation and treatment of menstrual disturbances is rarely needed, as the menstrual cycle will return to normal once binge eating, starvation, vomiting, excessive exercise, and abuse of laxatives have ceased. Investigation for polycystic ovarian syndrome (PCOS) is occasionally indicated.

Pregnancy may occasionally occur even if the woman has not started menstruating again (see Chapter 7, page 121). During the period of recovery from bulimia nervosa, many women need reassurance that they will not have become sterile as a result of their infrequent or absent ovulation and menstruation.

Fact!

If sexually active, the woman must use contraception to avoid an unwanted pregnancy.

Bulimia nervosa does not cause infertility.

Where should a patient with bulimia nervosa be treated?

When the diagnosis has been made and the patient's condition has been assessed, several approaches to treatment are available (see Chapter 6), and the advantages and disadvantages should be discussed by the therapist and the patient. The possibilities are:

◆ guided self-help;

◆ treatment as an outpatient;

◆ treatment as a day-patient or partial hospitalization;

◆ treatment as an inpatient.

These treatment options range from least to most supportive. Day-patient and inpatient treatment usually offer a combination of individual and group sessions with members of a multidisciplinary team, while outpatient treatment usually consists of individual sessions with the therapist, dietician, and other members of a multidisciplinary team as required.

Taking an individual approach to therapy allows treatment to be planned to meet the needs of an individual woman, her stage of illness, her current beliefs and attitudes, her motivation to change, and the external difficulties or stress factors that may be preventing her recovery. This may be why the CBT approach is thought to be slightly more effective if used for individuals rather than in group therapy.

Treatment in hospital has the advantage of enabling much to be accomplished in a short period of time. In most cases, hospital admission and inpatient treatment are not suggested in the first instance. The indications for inpatient treatment are given in the box below. Women who are admitted to hospital tend to have severe symptoms, or to have multiple psychological or physical problems. This may explain why hospital treatment seems to be no more successful than outpatient treatment in effecting a cure.

Possible reasons for admitting a patient with bulimia nervosa to hospital

- She is in poor physical health because she uses dangerous methods of weight control

- She has medical, or psychiatric problems that are best managed in hospital (for example, depression, drug dependence, personality disorder, diabetes)

- She is suicidal

- Her home environment is preventing changes in her eating behaviour

- Her personality is such that outpatient treatment is unlikely to be effective

- She lives in a rural or remote area where outpatient treatment is not available

- No improvement has been obtained following outpatient or day-patient treatment

- Her life is in crisis and she may benefit from a short stay in hospital

- She needs containment of her behaviour to allow assessment and to plan treatment

The problems and experiences of some women who require admission to hospital are graphically illustrated by extracts from the diary of a delightful 19-year-old patient, called Erin (see *Patient's perspective*). She used writing in her diary as a therapeutic tool.

 Patient's perspective

An extract from Erin's dairy:

Week one

First, I must accept the fact that it is my problem and, even if it isn't all my fault, I am the one who has to do the work to cure it . . . and not play games . . .

I need to give some time to myself to think about my problem. I have to stop trying to keep busy to stop trying to take my mind off the problem and to stop the loneliness.

I'm thinking about packing up and leaving and sorting it out at home instead of here ...

I want to know more about my problem:

—why has it happened?

—what happens to me?

—what I need to get better ... ?

I wish there were some rules to follow to get better, it's so hard because it is not a physical problem; it's emotional and psychological ...

The one cause or associated problem is my fear of being alone, which is pretty paradoxical. I'm afraid of being left alone because I know that I'll lose control and binge eat. On the other hand, when I'm feeling like binge eating, I get irritated when somebody is with me because they are preventing me from starting the binge. That is the paradox I'm beginning to understand ...

The anxieties that started me binge eating have long since passed I think. Now the binge eating is habitual and creates anxieties instead of the anxieties creating the binge. The anxieties that are created by the loss of control, and the binge, and the low self-esteem that goes with it, cause the binge-eating behaviour. I'm not sure how to correct this but think that it has some relevance—there's more to it as well I'm sure ...

End of week one

God, where do I start? I'm really so confused ... there's so much to grasp at once.

I'm constantly trying to please people and to do what I believe they expect of me and I have stopped being myself because of it. Always being ready to listen to and to help others. Always being selfless is partly a cause of this problem.

Week two

I've been very moody and restless since Wednesday. Woke up OK today but since breakfast I've been really angry. Stuffed myself with cereal and feel revolting and fat. Just want to throw it up—now I know that anger leads to purging: anger, self-disgust, revulsion and hatred ...

End of week two

Still angry and frustrated and confused. All day I felt dreadful ... felt fat and ugly and dreadfully alone and empty. I cried, not understanding what was going on. I was ultra-upset after my appointment with the dietician. She made it clear to me just how I've been stuffing myself around by cutting back on my menu plan. To cut back while being in here is stupid because the minute I go out I'll cut back, deny myself things and then binge and vomit and be back to square one. It's just so futile! All I want to do is lose weight and get over this eating disorder. I have to stop cutting back, which means stop losing weight ...

End of week three

I want to go home. But I know that's running away. But it won't really be running away. I'll be running away from this environment to another environment, but the feelings won't change. I can run away as far as possible, but I can't run away from how I'm feeling.

Oh, what a day! YUCK ... YUCK ... YUCK ... ! [Later] The best thing I did for myself tonight was to stop myself from binge eating and I feel so good about it.

End of week four

Some nights when I have the urge to binge I don't go near the kitchen. I feel strong and those times are positive. But tonight's defeat of the Bulimic Binge Devil was even stronger. Stronger because I'd taken the first step and there was no chance of being caught. And the best thing was that I did it for myself. For nobody else but me and I did it for me because I deserve to beat it.

Week five

Went home on Friday. Aaaaaaarghhhh! I'm going up and down like a yo-yo. It's unbelievable. I did vomit and then felt so guilty, mainly for Mum but also for myself.

End of week five

This morning I woke up with a new attitude. I realized last night that going home without taking responsibility just wasn't the answer. Responsibility for my own dilemma was the key to beating it. I made some decisions …

Spoke to my doctor which annoyed me because she emphasized the importance of getting on with it.

I can't FANTASIZE … I must do it.

If the woman has been treated in hospital and a day programme is available for 1 or 2 days a week, this may provide additional support during the transition from inpatient to outpatient therapy. A weekend programme can allow the woman to return to study or work immediately after leaving hospital.

 Fact!

It is best to go straight back to work or school after inpatient treatment.

A woman will find the transition much easier if she has to make only one change in her routine between being an inpatient and her normal daily pattern of living. For this reason, going on holiday or any temporary change in lifestyle or structure of the day between being in hospital and outpatient follow-up treatment is not recommended.

Response to treatment

'The binges still occur but I would define them now as "over-eating". My weight has gone up 3 kg (6½ lbs) but it doesn't bother me. I don't weigh myself anymore, at least not often. I don't try to stick to a diet as it would just emphasize food once again (but I'm sure that I will always count calories in my mind—but only in hundreds). I feel happy and try to eat normally whenever possible.'

A good response to treatment is where:

- the woman ceases to binge eat;

- she ceases to use potentially dangerous methods of weight control;

- her weight is stable;

- she eats regular meals;

- she is able to interact with others in social situations;

- her self-esteem is good and is not dependent on her image; and

- she has a good quality of life.

Relapse and relapse prevention

In the first 2 years of recovery from bulimia nervosa, women will experience urges to start binge eating or vomiting again. Relapses are common at this time and may last weeks or months. The urge is usually precipitated by a stressful situation: a change of job, illness, marriage, divorce, abortion, or the birth of a dead or deformed baby. The woman should contact her therapist to discuss her problems and put in place some of the relapse-prevention strategies in the box below.

Relapse prevention suggestions

If you want to binge, vomit, or starve yourself:

- keep eating in a structured pattern: three meals with snacks at similar times each day;

- think through your problem and try to find a way to overcome it, other than by binge eating or eating to vomit;

- talk about your problem with someone you can trust;

- learn your warning signs, e.g. feelings of anxiety, unease, or depression;

- learn what triggers these thoughts. e.g. an argument with a parent;

- practise ways you have learnt to cope with unpleasant and anxiety-provoking feelings;

- find enjoyable ways of resting and relaxing;

- try to keep yourself occupied and with people at times when you are likely to binge or vomit;

- remember the methods you used to 'resist' binge eating in the past and employ some of them;

- make sure you have not lost weight;

- do not weigh yourself; if you must, never more than once each week;

- make exercise enjoyable, non-stressful, and only one of many ways of coping with stress;

- plan ahead if going overseas or changing your lifestyle;

- keep in contact with your therapist.

ⓘ Patient's perspective

'Almost 5 years have passed since my second eating disorder episode. I have recognized that the way I have responded in the past to adverse changes in my life has not been very helpful. My first reaction was always to deny the change, to fight it entirely, even though deep down I must have known that fighting was futile and the change was inevitable. Hiding inside an eating disorder is really only a temporary solution, a coping mechanism and not a very good one at that. For over 15 years I lived in a world of constant anxiety, waiting for the next calamity to hit me, believing that somehow I deserved it. Sometimes you have to walk through a wall of fire to get where you want to be—or to get away from where you don't want to be. For me, the last episode was enough for me to make a conscious decision to change my life. I walked away from an unsatisfying life in a foreign country and a career that I no longer found interesting. I said goodbye to some of my dearest friends and returned to my home country with no real plan at all. Somehow it has all worked out. Shortly after returning to the city I grew up in, I landed a great job that I really enjoy. I met a wonderful man and we are now planning our future together. All in all I have to say that life is pretty good these days. I know that life will continue to deal savage blows but I believe I am better equipped to handle them now.'

Outcome of bulimia nervosa

 Patient's perspective

Yvonne described her life, 15 years after treatment:

'It's good to feel "normal" about eating and my weight now. I eat whatever I feel like, including cakes, an occasional chocolate, bread, ice cream, rich savoury dishes like quiche or pies. I eat when I want to, but I have found that I enjoy food most when I am hungry and can sit and eat leisurely. I have also found that my stomach will signal when it's full (although it's too easy to miss the signal at times) and I usually stop eating then. It's like regular people who eat when they're hungry and stop when they're full. My appetite varies tremendously. However, if I discover myself constantly in the kitchen searching for "something" simply to put in my mouth, I realize I am bored or uptight and am seeking a pacifier. Then, I ask myself, "Exactly what food would I like?" Often the answer comes back, "Well, nothing really," or "I don't know," and then (if I feel like it) I will say to myself, "You're not hungry really; you're just looking for a diversion," and go away to find something else to do.

My weight varies in cycles (this being deduced, not from the tyranny of the bathroom scales, but from the looseness of the clothes around my waist).

My weight does not worry me, nor do I try to control it by strict dieting. If I feel "heavy", I will eat less food and drink less, watch for that point of stomach fullness, and exercise more.

There are cycles of heaviness when I feel heavy and have been overeating. It's nice to know the connection between weight and eating. I know when I am eating more and I feel my weight going up—not like before when I always seemed "fat" regardless of how much or how little I ate.

Then there are slim cycles when I feel slimmer, trimmer, and eat less, but this just happens and I do not control it or feel guilty about eating less or more ...

Recently, under much pressure of work and relationships, I started experiencing a "knot" in my stomach. It immediately reminded me of my binge-days when I often had this knot and thought it was hunger. Then, I would eat to relieve the "hunger". Food soothed away the pain and did, in fact, make me feel "better", no longer being plagued by a gnawing in the stomach. However, when I ate food or drank milk to relieve the knot, it relieved it temporarily but then left me in 5 minutes again feeling the same. It was a tension build-up and I learnt I could relieve it by deep breaths (trying to relax) or walking around and stretching. It went away after a couple of weeks.'

Table 10.2 Outcome of bulimia nervosa after 10–15 years

Outcome	%
Cured	50
Intermediate[a]	30
Poor[b]	20

[a] Features of an eating disorder consistent with women in the community who 'watch their weight'.

[b] Still suffering from bulimia nervosa, an 'eating disorder not otherwise specified', or binge-eating disorder.

It is important for the patient and her family to know what the long-term outcome of bulimia nervosa is. At present, three long-term studies over a period of 10–15 years have been reported, including one involving our own patients. The results of all three studies are very similar and are from the UK, USA, and Australia (see Table 10.2).

Women with a 'poor' outcome 10–15 years after the first presentation binge ate less frequently than they had done previously and most seldom or no longer induced vomiting or purged. It appears that, for some women, there may be a continuum from bulimia nervosa through to binge-eating disorder to recovery. None of the patients had anorexia nervosa. Some women stop their bulimic behaviour only to replace it with an exercise disorder or alcohol dependence. They should not be considered recovered. Mortality is around 1–2%, with suicide being the most common reason for death.

The 30% of women who had some features of, or behaviour associated with, an eating disorder after 10–15 years resembled 'normal' women who are concerned about their body shape and weight. These 'normal' women may have occasional episodes of binge eating or food restriction, but these episodes do not interfere with the woman's quality of life. Such women have been identified in the community as 'restrained eaters'.

Factors predicting outcome

Factors predicting a good outcome of treatment are as follows:

◆ treatment is sought early;

◆ the woman has not had episodes of anorexia nervosa (been at low body weight);

◆ the woman has not induced vomiting;

- the woman has not been at high body weight before or during treatment;

- there are no co-morbid psychological, psychiatric, or medical problems;

- the woman has not had close relatives treated for psychiatric problems, such as depression, alcohol dependency, or anxiety disorders.

Summary of the treatment of bulimia nervosa

Treatment takes place as an outpatient, day-patient, or inpatient.

Help the patient to:

- stop trying to lose weight;

- stop using weight-losing behaviour;

- learn sensible, normal eating patterns, appropriate to their lifestyle;

- eat at least three meals and two or three snacks each day (structured eating);

- decrease their preoccupation with weight and food;

- gain confidence about eating normally and not gaining weight.

Throughout the programme provide:

- supportive psychotherapy including crisis intervention when needed;

- cognitive behaviour and other psychological therapies;

- help for other perceived problems;

- assistance in improving self-esteem.

Once binge eating and weight-losing behaviours have ceased, if the woman is still overweight and wishes to lose weight, sensible supervised dieting may be attempted. However, dieting is usually not necessary as a slow, persistent weight loss occurs over a period of months or years.

The overall aim is to help the patient:

- to live a normal life;

- to be able to cope with life (be resilient).

11

Investigation and treatment of obesity and overeating disorders

→ Key points

- Modest decreases in weight can make significant improvements to health

- The four main treatment components are: participation in regular exercise, acceptance of a menu plan, learning new eating behaviours, and making lifestyle changes to ensure the changes can be maintained

- Sensible healthy weight loss is slow and sometimes non-existent; weight maintenance with no disordered behaviours should be accepted as progress.

- Supportive psychotherapy with cognitive behaviour and other psychological techniques help modify unhelpful thoughts and behaviours

- Drugs can be used in the treatment of obesity to support the person trying to implement the four abovementioned components; they should not replace other treatments

- Bariatric surgery is considered for persons with a BMI of >35 with medical and psychological sequelae

'My other good news is that my weight isn't such a worry any more. I am still overweight, but I certainly don't feel the grotesque elephant I used to feel. I'm a BMI of 28 at the moment, which is low for me, and I haven't put on any weight for about 7 months. I'm not really dieting I guess . . . just eating pretty sensibly and that seems to be enough to keep my weight stable. I know it's a slow and black way to lose weight, but this way my eating doesn't dominate my thoughts so much.'

Obesity in the general population

Obesity is one of the major health problems of this century. The prevalence of overweight and obese people is rising rapidly in Europe, the USA, Australia and some parts of Asia and South America. Obesity is associated with a poor quality of life, significant morbidity, and premature death. It is predicted that teenagers entering adulthood with a BMI of 40 or more will have their life expectancy reduced by up to 13 years for males and 8 years for females.

Aims of treatment

The aims of the treatment of obesity are:

◆ to commence regular, enjoyable exercise;

◆ to learn to eat according to a sensibly chosen menu plan;

◆ to learn 'normal' structured eating behaviour;

◆ to acquire new attitudes to food and eating;

◆ to make lifestyle changes to help prevent weight gain in the future;

◆ to acquire skills to change unhelpful thoughts and behaviours;

◆ to help improve self-esteem;

◆ to provide support and reassurance.

Investigation of obesity

The patient's history should explore any possible reasons why the person is obese. Questions should be asked in a sensitive manner and the health professional should recognize that there is growing support and acceptance of obesity in the community. Some people visit a health professional merely to be reassured that, even though they are overweight or obese, they are healthy.

Measuring body fat

Body mass index (BMI, kg/m^2) is used to assess obesity (see Chapter 2) and measurement of waist circumference may also be included. BMI is the most useful clinical measure and is easy to calculate from the weight and height of the person. However, BMI can be slightly inaccurate in very fit and muscular men as they weigh 'heavy' and in elderly people who have lost muscle mass and who weigh 'light'.

Physical examination

The physical examination needs to be thorough and the doctor will assess each obese person for early signs or the presence of the following medical problems, which are associated with obesity:

- Type 2 diabetes
- Coronary heart disease
- Hypertension
- Gall bladder disease
- Obstructive sleep apnoea
- Depression
- Dyslipidaemia (elevation of lipids in the blood)
- Osteoarthritis (inflammation and pain in weight-bearing joints)
- Polycystic ovarian syndrome
- Steatohepatitis (accumulation of fat in the liver)
- Cancer (breast, uterus, prostate, colon).

Polycystic ovarian syndrome is a hormonal disturbance associated with irregular menstruation, reduced fertility, and sometimes acne and increased hairiness due to increases in male hormones. While the causes are unknown, insulin resistance, diabetes, and obesity are all strongly correlated with this syndrome. It may also be more common among women with bulimia nervosa.

Laboratory tests

The blood tests, including biochemical and hormonal investigations, that are carried out will depend on the patient's history, the result of the physical examination, and recent behaviours. The test may include blood glucose, triglycerides, cholesterol, thyroid function, measures of liver and kidney function, nutritional status, and electrolytes (see Chapter 5).

History

The history of the person's eating behaviour should be investigated as suggested in Chapter 5, and enquiries should be made to find out whether the person binge eats, has periods of strict dieting interspersed with binge eating, eats only at night, eats only once a day, 'grazes' throughout the day, or has other disordered eating patterns.

Suggestion: Try to think of times when your weight was stable for 3 months or more without dieting.

Other aspects that should be addressed in the medical history include the medications the patient is taking and her alcohol consumption, smoking habits, and use of recreational drugs. If the person is female, her menstrual and reproductive history should be reviewed. The history includes inquiring about any family history of obesity and looking for a possible hormonal or other physical and psychological causes for her body weight.

Psychological assessment

The aim of this assessment is to find out why the person has sought help at this time. Most obese people have been overweight for months or years before seeking help. When the person seeks help, usually something has happened to precipitate their concern about being obese. It may be that the person has been consistently teased about their appearance, or has been prodded to seek help by a close person, or that their health has worsened. A desire for pregnancy or intimacy, or a breakdown in a close relationship may stimulate women to seek help. Their story should be listened to and emotions such as sadness, disappointment, or overconcern should be addressed at the same time as treatment is offered.

Treatment of obesity

Weight loss is not easy and those people who decide to try to lose weight and maintain the weight loss can be helped by four complementary strategies: regular exercise, following a menu plan, learning 'normal' eating, and making modifications to lifestyle that ensure that these changes in eating and behaviour can be maintained. 'Normal' eating is discussed in Chapter 10.

 Fact!

Cognitive behaviour therapy can help modify unhelpful beliefs and behaviours.

The psychological approaches available for the treatment of eating disorders (see Chapter 6) should be discussed with the woman and her individual needs addressed. A basic supportive psychotherapeutic and cognitive behaviour therapy approach (see Chapter 10) will probably be recommended in the first instance. Other psychological techniques, such as mindfulness and mindful eating, can be included as appropriate. Individual and groups approaches will be recommended.

Exercise

Regular exercise aids weight loss, although the degree to which it helps seems to vary from person to person. Men, with their greater muscle mass, will lose weight faster than women for a given amount of exercise. The approximate amount of time you have to exercise to use up a certain amount of energy is shown in Table 11.1.

Different exercise regimens have different benefits. Jogging, for example, puts stress on joints, which swimming does not. Swimming has the disadvantage that the body is supported by the water and less energy is burnt off. Probably the best, most efficient, and least damaging exercise is walking, but in choosing

Table 11.1 Energy expenditure of certain physical activities

Activity	Average time (in minutes) required to burn off different amounts of energy		
	Energy burnt off:		
	400 kJ	800 kJ	1200 kJ
Walking, golf (21 kJ per min)	19	36	57
Cycling, tennis, swimming (30 kJ per min)	13	26	40
Jogging (42 kJ per min)	9	19	28

an exercise programme, the person should choose one or more than one, that most appeals to them.

 Fact!

Exercise must be regular—preferably daily—and the frequency and duration of time spent exercising should be increased gradually.

Having a pedometer and aiming for 10,000 steps each day can be helpful.

Weight-reducing programmes

Fad diets do not work. Many diets have been devised, and many have failed to produce either the desired weight loss or to enable the person to maintain the new lower weight permanently. A few strictly controlled very-low-energy diets help very obese people to start losing weight, and are successful in the short term, but do not provide a balanced regimen that is a long-term option. These very restrictive diets may be offered if the person is highly motivated to lose weight, for example so that they can have surgery. These should only be attempted under strict medical supervision, as they can cause life-threatening conditions and even death.

 Fact!

The woman needs to learn new eating behaviours that are not perceived as 'dieting' but rather as 'normal eating', which will continue after weight has been lost.

Weight loss is a slow process and the person will need help. The support, information, and encouragement offered by self-help groups such as Weight Watchers, and from a psychologist, physician, or dietician will enhance the patient's motivation, encourage new skills, and offer help in dealing with situations that may be associated with the urge to eat excessively.

Slow rather than rapid weight loss

It is important to know that an average loss of weight of 0.5–1.0 kg (1–2 lb) is the maximum usually obtained after the first few weeks (when a weight loss of 2–4 kg (4–8 lb) a week may occur) and the most appropriate programmes are designed to help the person achieve this small but steady loss of weight. However, as in the treatment of anorexia nervosa and bulimic nervosa, a menu plan alone is not enough; motivation to resist the urge to eat and to keep to the programme is equally essential.

In the first weeks of a severe reducing diet, or of starvation, a quick weight loss may be expected as the energy in the glycogen–water pool is used up and a large quantity of water is lost to the body. However, the energy in the pool will be depleted within 1–4 weeks. After this time, any further weight loss has to come from 'burning up' the adipose tissue to release energy. The second component of weight loss is a slow, steady loss. The amount lost weekly will depend on the restriction of energy intake, but rarely exceeds 0.5–1.0 kg (1–2 lb) per week.

A further problem when a person loses weight is that their metabolic rate slows down. The consequence of this is that, even if a person tries to lose weight and sticks with the weight-reducing programme, the weight loss may stop for a time. At that point, the person needs support and should not be accused of failing to adhere to their programme.

 ## Patient's perspective

'It all started about 10 years ago, at a time when many things in my family's and my life were pretty tough. I felt that I was everybody's prop and couldn't escape. I wasn't aware at first that my weight began to rise, until I found I needed a size 16 dress instead of a size 12. I tried to diet but the problems remained and food seemed to be the only way I could dull the pain. I got into the habit of looking in the mirror, being depressed at what I saw, and eating some more so that I could cope. I dieted and began losing weight, and then I'd give it up and eat enormous amounts and gain weight once more.

My behaviour became destructive to me. I now know I was using food as an escape from emotional pain and stress. I was really no different from an alcoholic, and I realized I wasn't going to conquer it alone, but there was nowhere to go. I was on a roller coaster of eating and dieting and I couldn't get off. I didn't induce vomiting or take laxatives or anything like that. It wasn't as if I had thought of these things and rejected them—I hadn't even thought of them.

I knew I had an eating disorder. I wasn't in control of food but food was controlling me. I was a fat girl and I wanted to be thin, but I couldn't keep to a diet to become thin. I'm still a fat girl. I wish I could get thinner.'

The menu plan and weight reduction

It is best to consult a dietician about a menu plan that is suited to your needs. The principles of the menu plan are that it should:

◆ supply less than the person's energy requirements;

◆ consist of three meals and two or three snacks each day;

◆ provide a wide variety of foods;

◆ provide all nutrient requirements except energy;

◆ be acceptable to the person;

◆ be able to be sustained;

◆ fit in with the family meals;

◆ be compatible with social eating;

◆ not impair health or well-being (e.g. low-fibre diets may cause constipation);

◆ allow a good quality of life.

The dietician and a support group will also remind people about the following principles of a weight-losing menu, outlined in the box below.

General rules of a weight-losing menu plan

◆ Eat lean meat (e.g. poultry) without the skin

◆ Grill food instead of frying

◆ Spread butter/margarine thinly

◆ Avoid energy-dense foods not included in your menu plan

◆ Reduce the amount of sugar added to tea, coffee, or cereals

◆ Be aware of the sugars in fruit juices and other drinks

◆ Limit the intake of alcohol

The menu plan and disordered eating

A menu plan can also be used to help stabilize disordered eating behaviours and prevent further weight gain. This menu plan has all the principles of the previous one except the energy provided is normal for an average weight person of the same height, age, and sex. Along with psychological therapy, this approach will maximize the chances of ceasing eating-disordered behaviour, prevent further weight gain, and usually produces a small steady weight loss. This is the idea behind the 'stop dieting and lose weight' approach to weight reduction. In other words, if you eliminate the drive to eat resulting from undereating, when you are obese, you will lose weight.

 Fact!

Weight stabilization is a major achievement.

Aiming to eat a 'normal weight' menu plan will:

◆ stop feelings of failure;

◆ prevent feelings of hunger and deprivation;

◆ teach good sustainable eating habits;

◆ help control disordered eating behaviour, e.g. binge eating;

◆ have a long-term side effect of weight loss (very slow).

 Fact!

An obese woman will lose weight if she eats a normal menu plan that would maintain her weight if she had a normal BMI.

Behavioural strategies

Learning new eating behaviours

 Fact!

A menu plan, in itself, will not enable a person to lose weight, however carefully it is devised.

In order to follow a menu plan the person must be motivated to structure each day, to keep to the plan, and to understand what is involved. Motivation can be encouraged in several ways, and the most appropriate way for each person should be chosen. Many people find that their motivation to lose weight is increased if they can share experiences with and obtain support from other people also trying to lose weight. The support needs to extend throughout the period of weight reduction. Support is also needed when the person has achieved the lower weight, so that she does not regain weight swiftly or insidiously.

There can be weeks of almost no weight loss measured on the scales. During this time, it is easy for people to lose their motivation and 'give up'. Counselling about how the body responds to food deprivation, variations in metabolic rate, and fluid changes is important and reassuring during weight loss.

The following is a list of some suggested changes that can help to achieve a successful weight loss:

1. *Keep active and take more planned exercise.* Find enjoyable activities. Don't do exercise you hate. It is helpful if you go for a walk, or do something active, after a meal. This is because exercise induces heat production and energy loss.

2. *Don't go on a 'crash' diet.* Initially these diets produce a rapid weight loss (water), but it is very hard to keep to them and overeating usually follows. If a crash diet and semi-starving persists for a month, the body reacts by reducing the basal metabolic rate, so that less energy is burned up than if eating a sensible weight-reducing diet. In fact, the body becomes more efficient at storing fat.

3. *Don't weigh yourself more than once each week.* It is tempting to eat more if your weight goes down, and to become despondent, lose motivation, and eat more when it goes up. Weight fluctuates from day to day depending on many variables including the fluid balance of the body.

4. *Choose a menu plan that is nutritious and is sufficiently varied and tasty to enable you to stick to it without getting bored or frustrated.* Low glycaemic index carbohydrates and a certain amount of protein and essential fatty acids from fish and nuts should be part of the diet. The menu plan should also contain sufficient vitamins, minerals, and dietary fibre to keep you in good health. Each meal should look attractive, smell pleasant, and taste good so that the meal is enjoyed.

5. *Do not limit the dietary fibre in your food.* The result may be constipation, and the risk of developing cancer of the large bowel, coronary heart disease, and haemorrhoids is increased.

6. *Don't gorge by eating only one large meal a day.* Weight will be lost more quickly if several small meals spread out over the day are eaten. No meal should be skipped and the last meal should not be just before going to bed. Smaller meals eaten at shorter intervals induce a greater production of body heat, which is then dissipated into the surrounding air. Body heat is produced using energy, which is burned up from the body. Eating more often prevents binge eating.

7. *Try to eat sitting at a table and use utensils when you eat.* Distractions such as watching TV, reading, or walking about when eating will lead to more food being eaten.

8. *Meals should be at similar times each day.* This helps the physiological and psychological control of hunger and satiation.

9. *Eat slowly when you have a meal.* Wait until your mouth is empty before you take the next bite. Eating slowly and chewing meticulously teaches people to be satisfied with less food and to enjoy the smaller quantity more. This is called 'mindful eating'.

10. *Decide beforehand the amount of food you are going to put on your plate.* Picking leads to weight gain.

11. *Stop eating as soon as you feel full, no matter what is left on the plate.* This helps to break the habit of continuing to eat until all of the food has gone.

12. *Leave the table once you feel full or have finished your meal (if you can do so without offending anyone).* Staying at the table where there is food may break the resolve not to eat any more.

13. *Do not eat other people's leftovers.* Children can leave a lot of food over a day. Put the leftovers in the bin or into a container in the freezer to make soup at a later date.

14. *Don't keep a store of sweets, biscuits, chocolate, chips, or nuts in the house or office.* It is easier to resist the temptation to nibble when bored or unhappy if they are not there.

15. *Don't take food with you when you go out.* Although you may feel uncomfortable at first, this will pass. Getting in touch with your feelings and learning that they will pass is part of getting better.

16. *Only go shopping for food when you have eaten.* People react less to the sight of food when they are not hungry. Only food that is needed should be bought (have a list). It is also helpful to buy food that needs to be prepared, rather than a tin or packet that only needs to be opened.

17. *Don't be 'conned' into choosing a complicated or expensive diet.* You will not keep to it. Choose a menu plan that can be used for life.

Drugs in the management of obesity

The role of drugs in the management of obesity is currently seen as an adjunct to the core treatments of dietary counselling, supportive psychotherapy, and other psychological therapies aimed at modifying eating-related activities and beliefs, exercise to increase energy expenditure, and menu plans to lower food intake. Anti-obesity drugs should only be used in combination with these methods.

Currently, only two drugs are used to treat obesity, sibutramine and orlistat. The prescribing guidelines for the use of anti-obesity drugs recommend a BMI of 30 or more or a 'co-morbid condition', such as high blood pressure, diabetes, or hyperlipidaemia. The drugs have different actions. Sibutramine enhances satiety and reduces the desire to eat, while orlistat acts on the gut to reduce fat being absorbed into the body. The newest drug showing promise in current trials is rimonabant, an endocannabinoid receptor antagonist that acts on the cells of the hypothalamus, a region of the brain where appetite is controlled (see Chapter 2). This drug is promising because it appears to result in weight loss over a longer period of time. It was initially trialled to help with the cessation of smoking, but was found to be better for weight loss.

Sibutramine

Sibutramine is a monoamine reuptake inhibitor, a drug that alters serotonin and noradrenaline (neurotransmitters) in the brain. As with other drugs of this nature, the side effects of dry mouth, constipation, agitation, and insomnia may be a nuisance. This drug should only be taken with medical supervision and may not be suitable for all obese people, particularly those with blood pressure problems, as it may increase blood pressure and pulse rate in some people. This is the first drug of this kind to be used in the treatment of obesity and the long-term effects of taking this drug are unknown at this time. Accompanied by a menu plan, a weight loss of 10 kg (22 lb) may be maintained for at least 2 years. This is twice the weight loss achieved with a meal plan and placebo tablets.

Orlistat

Orlistat is a gastrointestinal lipase inhibitor, i.e. it decreases the amount of fat absorbed from the gut. To enable fat to be absorbed by the body, it must first be broken down into fatty acids and glycerol by the enzyme lipase in the small intestine (see page 208). When eating a meal containing fat and taking a lipase inhibitor, the fat is not broken down and fatty and oily stools are passed. In fact, eating a fatty meal is not very pleasant as it can result in a lot of flatulence (gas), very smelly and fatty diarrhoea, urgency, and sometimes incontinence. Because of these unpleasant side effects, people learn to reduce the amount of fat they eat and even learn to avoid 'hidden fats'. In this way, lipase inhibitors reduce energy intake and change people's eating behaviour and food selection. As vitamins A and D are absorbed into our body dissolved in fat, a few people may become deficient in these essential vitamins. Orlistat and sibutramine are equally effective at weight reduction.

 Fact!

Even modest weight losses of 5–10% produce significant improvements in the risk factors associated with obesity.

Weight loss surgery

Bariatric or weight loss surgery should not be seen as a 'quick fix' for gross obesity. It should only be offered by a team of professionals who manage obesity and who can provide the necessary medical, dietetic, and psychological preparation and follow-up. The indications for surgery are that the person has a BMI over 35 kg/m^2, has identifiable medical or psychological problems associated with their obesity, and all other attempts at weight loss have failed. Below a BMI of 35 kg/m^2, the seriousness of the medical problem must greatly outweigh the risk of the operation before a person would be considered for the operation. The surgical procedures currently recommended in the treatment for obesity surgery are adjustable gastric banding, gastric bypass, and bilopancreatic diversion. Adjustable gastric banding is now performed most often and is the first choice for many people.

Before the operation takes place, the patient must undergo a thorough physical examination and psychological assessment, and must be fully informed of the risks and possible complications of the operation. The type of operation and the reasons for the operation will be explained, and this will include the anatomy of the gastrointestinal tract and the physiology of digestion.

Physiology of digestion

The primary function of the digestive tract is to provide the body with a continual supply of water, electrolytes, and nutrients. This is achieved by (1) movement of the food through the oesophagus, stomach, and intestines; (2) secretion of

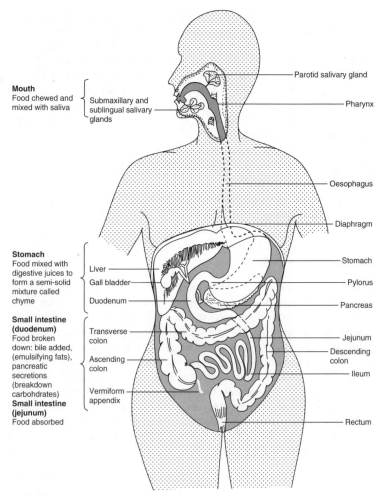

Figure 11.1 The intestinal tract

digestive juices; and (3) absorption of the digested foods, water, and electrolytes from the intestines.

The movement and mixing of foods occurs because slowly-moving peristaltic waves of contractions pass regularly along the alimentary tract in response to its distension by food or water. These contractions squeeze the food onwards, mixing it at the same time. In the mouth, food is masticated and mixed with saliva. It is then swallowed and passes through the oesophagus to enter the stomach. The stomach can store large quantities of food until it can be accommodated in the intestine. During its period in the stomach, the food is mixed with gastric digestive juices and dilute hydrochloric acid to form a semi-fluid mixture and is partially broken down. As space becomes available in the intestines, this mixture, called chyme, is moved from the stomach by peristaltic waves of contractions.

Most of the absorption of food takes place in the small intestine where the chyme is acted on by secretions from the gall bladder and pancreas, and other intestinal digestive juices. Fats are emulsified by the action of bile salts and digested by secretions from the pancreas and intestines. In this state, they are absorbed by the intestines, and the greater the distension of the intestines, the greater is the absorption.

An understanding of these physiological concepts led to the idea that if most of the small intestine was bypassed the patient would be able to eat but would lose weight because the food would not be absorbed. A second idea, which was developed somewhat later after the complications following bypass surgery became apparent, was to reduce the size of the stomach. It was argued that if the size of the stomach was reduced by two-thirds or more, the patient would be prevented from eating large meals because a feeling of fullness (satiety) would occur after small meals.

Gastric bypass

The gastric bypass, also called a Roux-en-Y gastric bypass, is the oldest surgical method for weight reduction. The idea of this operation is to bypass the main part of the stomach and parts of the small intestine to reduce the area in which food is reabsorbed. This is achieved by separating the upper part of the stomach from the main part. The small intestine is also cut and then attached by one end directly to the upper part of the stomach. The other end is sutured to the part of the small intestine coming down from the stomach, building a Y-shaped loop (Figure 11.2). On average, 50–60% of the excess weight is lost in the first 5 years after the operation. The main complications of this operation are shown in the box below.

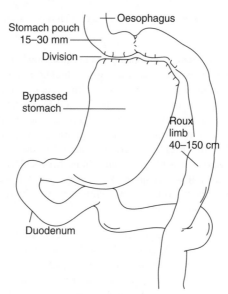

Figure 11.2 A Roux-en-Y gastric bypass

Complications and undesirable side effects of gastric bypass surgery

- Wound complications (leakage)

- Bowel obstruction

- Gastrointestinal tract haemorrhage

- Pulmonary embolus

- Wound infection

- Pneumonia

- Incisional hernia

- Vitamin and mineral deficiencies (vitamins A, D, E, and B12, folate and iron)

- Gallstones

The complication rate is lower when the operation is conducted as a laparo-scopic procedure (keyhole surgery), which is possible when the person is not severely obese. As it is the quantity of food that produces the feeling of satiation, an unmotivated person can cheat by eating or drinking small amounts of energy-dense liquids or food, most of which is absorbed.

Bilopancreatic diversion

The idea of this operation is similar to a gastric bypass—to bypass part of the small intestines and also to have the bile and pancreatic digestive 'juices' entering the small intestine close to the site where it joins the colon, to give little time for the breakdown and absorption of fats. Once it has entered the colon, food is no longer absorbed back into the body.

Adjustable gastric bands

In this operation, an inflatable silicon band is put around the upper part of the stomach, leaving a tiny stomach pouch (Figure 11.3). This lap band is connected to a tube, which has a port on its far end that is placed under the skin. From this access port, the band can be inflated (tightened) or loosened by injecting or removing the saline solution in the tube and lap band (Figure 11.3). The band can be adjusted at any time.

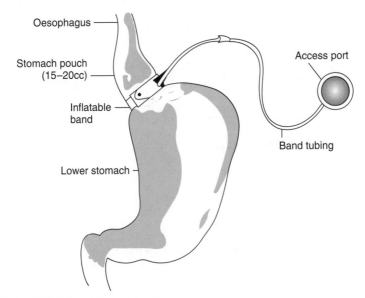

Figure 11.3 Adjustable gastric banding

The effect of gastric banding is that the person feels 'full' after eating a small amount of food, because the small pouch is stretched and messages are sent to the hypothalamus in the brain. Unless the patient eats slowly and keeps the amount small, the pouch will fill and additional food will remain in the oesophagus, leading to heartburn or vomiting. As both are uncomfortable, the patient learns to reduce their food intake and consequently loses weight.

As with any method, patients can cheat. Patients can binge eat large amounts of food and then vomit. They can develop bulimia nervosa. Others eat soft high-energy food and liquid that easily passes through.

Complications after a gastric band can be the development of gallstones, asymptomatic reflux and a hiatal hernia (where parts of the stomach prolapse through the band). Following gastric banding, patients lose weight rapidly: approximately 50–60% of excess weight is lost in the first 5 years.

There are a number of advantages of this method of weight loss, as described in the box below.

Advantages of adjustable lap banding compared with other bariatric surgery methods

- Less invasive—can be done by laparoscopy

- Reduced recovery time

- Reversible—the stomach regains its normal shape if removed, as nothing is cut

- Can be adjusted for pregnancy

- Safer, with a lower mortality

- Controllable and adjustable

- Fewer side effects

- Equally effective after 5 years

- Results in substantial improvement in the patient's quality of life

---

Counselling and support before and after surgery

Before the operation, the patient must clearly understand that the creation of a smaller stomach during surgery, which can last up to 1–2 hours, will not cure a psychological dependence on food or alter disordered eating habits. The patient must also be aware that, following the operation, vitamin and mineral supplements are necessary and pain may occur, as may episodes of diarrhoea, and appropriate follow-up, including blood tests, is essential. Patients should consider surgery as an adjunct to weight loss and not a substitute for sensible eating and exercise.

After bariatric surgery, dietetic counselling and education in nutrition is required, as a new eating behaviour has to be learnt. The essentials of good nutrition will again be emphasized and patients are also taught how to cope with a greatly diminished gastric reservoir, about the need to chew the food slowly and thoroughly, and the consequences that can occur (mainly vomiting) if they don't. They are also taught not to drink during meals as the food can swell up and not to drink anything cold before eating (see *Patient's perspective*: Diane).

 Patient's perspective

Diane, aged 55, has had both types of surgery.

She was brought up in a family with an abundance of food and feelings of being loved by her parents. Food was bought in bulk, never as single items. There were five well-stocked refrigerators in the home. Both her parents drank excessive amounts of alcohol and were seldom at home. Her father, who became jealous and violent when he had been drinking, drank at the local pub, while her mother frequented the more upmarket clubs. Diane was the eldest of seven children and was responsible for bringing up the five after herself. She was expected to go straight home from school every day to look after them. She left home when her mother became pregnant with the seventh child.

Diane described herself as 'chubby as a baby and always overweight' and felt that being overweight at school 'was the least of my problems'. At school, she was teased for being dirty and 'smelling bad' and was asked to sit away from the other children in the classroom. She had only one school uniform and one dress to wear to church each Sunday. The house was always chaotic, untidy, and dirty, and washing was only done episodically. In many ways, the children were neglected.

As she was growing up, Diane sometimes liked being overweight and act-ing 'rough' to annoy her mother who dressed well, was slim, and acted in a ladylike manner. To escape from home at 19 years, she asked for an inter-state transfer of her job. After she had left home, she enjoyed her life and was popular with friends and had boyfriends until she married at 30. She lost weight during a holiday when she was 19, and reached what she felt was a normal weight and felt she looked lovely (BMI of 28). At work, she is very conscientious and has always been in great demand. Over the years, her weight gradually increased to a BMI of 41, at the age of 33, when she became pregnant with her first child. She felt she had tried every popu-lar diet recommended by magazines and doctors, acupuncture, multiple medications prescribed by doctors, participation in clubs and weight-loss groups on many occasions, and had attended exercise groups and gyms.

When she was pregnant, she gave up smoking and stopped drinking, although she seldom drank alcohol. She felt she was a very disciplined person and couldn't understand why she couldn't stop eating.

In the year following the birth of her son, she reached a BMI of 50. She failed to become pregnant again and sought help for her infertility. In desperation, she agreed to an operation to reduce the length of her small intestine. A weight loss of 50 kg (98 lb) occurred over the following 12–18 months. She then became pregnant at once and was delighted by the birth of a healthy baby daughter. Two years after surgery, her weight gradually began to increase back to her present weight.

It was 20 years of chronic diarrhoea, wind pain . . . I hated going to the toilet—the pain was so bad, the smell was awful, and I had bacterial infec-tions so had to take tablets. I had it reversed 6 months ago and had a lap-band inserted.

I've been successful at everything I have set out to do except lose weight. When I have problems, I always think I deserve something—the only thing I want is food. Recently a dietician asked me to list things I find comforting. I could not think of anything except food—it is my comfort and my reward.

Diane buys in bulk and hoards food. She fears feeling hungry and always has food with her. Nowadays, she will take two pieces of fruit with her if she is driving somewhere; previously, this would have been two bags of sweets. To stop herself buying food, especially cakes, she has given large amounts of money to people collecting for charities in shopping centres. Binge eating is very rare and the two occasions of feeling urgently compelled to get food and eat were related to external stressful events. It is possible that Diane would binge eat more often if she did not always keep food with her.

Until the last 2 years when she started to develop knee problems because of the excess weight, Diane considered the worst feature of being over-weight was embarrassing her children. A child at pre-school asked her daughter if her mother was pregnant or just fat. Although she always dressed well, she felt she should not attend her children's school func-tions as her children might be humiliated. The rest of the time, she felt she successfully maintained the myth of the fat and happy girl who was fun-loving and joined in everything. She felt good about herself when she could do things for others and please them.

Although it is early days, the lap band is improving her self-esteem. She knows she is losing weight and she is attending a weight-control clinic (included as part of the surgery) each week. She is following what she has been advised and is being encouraged to do this by her clinic dieticians and surgeon—not to drink before, during, or for 30 minutes after meals as the food can swell up and get stuck, and not to drink anything cold before eating as it can make the stoma (hole) smaller, which makes it dif-ficult to eat. The other advice is to exercise.

'I can now walk the whole length of the shopping centre without sitting down and I can swim over 600 metres in 30 minutes. I wish I could bottle up the good feeling I have when I have exercised and eaten well—if only I could feel this when I am tempted to eat too much yogurt.'

Suction lipectomy (liposuction)

Liposuction is not a method in terms of classic obesity surgery, but is an operation that is often carried out in less-obese persons who have unwanted fat deposits on different parts of their body. These fat deposits cannot be removed by exercise or diet and so liposuction is used to 'shape' the body.

Liposuction should be done by an experienced surgeon and a trained assistant. The fatty tissue is infiltrated with a fluid consisting of a mixture of saline and local anaesthetic. After a certain time, a cannula is inserted into the area and the fatty tissue is sucked out through the cannula. The patient is awake during the operation and the position of the cannula has to be changed several times to make sure the area is reached from different angles to achieve the best cosmetic results. Following surgery, a compression bandage is wrapped firmly around the area. It may be painful and uncomfortable for some days and it may take 3–4 months for the final cosmetic result to be seen.

Benefits of weight reduction

In grossly obese people, surgery can be the first step in a weight-reducing process that includes a sensible planned menu plan and exercise programme. However, the advantages and disadvantages of the operation should be considered and discussed with the surgeon, dietician, and psychologist beforehand. Follow-up for some months after the operation must include sessions with the dietician and psychologist.

In spite of many potential problems of using surgery to treat gross obesity, such as the dangers of the operation, the complications that may follow surgery, the need for careful attention to diet, and for vitamin and mineral supplements, and the need for frequent follow-up visits, there is no doubt of the benefits of weight reduction following surgery. As many as 50–75% of patients will no longer have type 2 diabetes, high blood pressure, elevated blood lipid levels, fatty liver, or depression. There is an improvement in pulmonary ventilation, with a reduction in shortness of breath. If the person has osteoarthritis or low back pain, the severity of the pain is reduced. Following a significant reduction in weight, patients report that they feel more energetic and less fatigued.

The psychological benefits of surgery to achieve weight reduction have been less clearly delineated. As weight loss progresses, most patients perceive their bodies more favourably and become more confident. The majority of people see themselves as more sexually attractive; they experience fewer mood changes and see themselves as more self-assured, outgoing, and comfortable. They become more sociable, less preoccupied with their weight, and less likely to eat more than they intended at meals or between meals.

 Fact!

Following bariatric surgery, the quality of life scores (using question-naires) are no different to non-obese men and women.

Summary of the treatment of obesity

Treatment usually takes place as an outpatient.

The aim of treatment is to help the patient to:

- choose a sensible menu plan that reduces energy intake;

- eat at least three structured meals a day plus snacks;

- learn that the eating plan is for life and must be continued after weight loss;

- learn that long-term weight management is about enjoyable, realistic eating and exercise;

- be active and exercise regularly;

- modify unhelpful attitudes and behaviours;

- be motivated to continue, even when there is no weight loss;

- make changes in her lifestyle to support continued weight loss and weight maintenance.

Throughout treatment, the following should be provided:

- help for disordered eating;

- supportive psychotherapy;

- cognitive behaviour and other psychological therapies;

- help for other problems.

If the measures for treating mild or moderate obesity fail, seek the expertise of a multidisciplinary obesity team to discuss using:

- a very low energy diet (short intervention only);

- anti-obesity medications;

- adjustable gastric banding in conjunction with sensible eating and exercise, and continued follow-up and treatment from the multidisciplinary team.

The overall aim is:

- to improve the person's quality of life.

Appendix A

Body mass index (BMI) charts and height conversion

BMI CHARTS

Height (ft-in)	Height (m)	Height² (m²)	BMI 17 (kg)	BMI 18 (kg)	BMI 19 (kg)	BMI 20 (kg)	BMI 25 (kg)	BMI 30 (kg)	BMI 35 (kg)	BMI 40 (kg)
	1.45	2.10	35.70	37.80	40.00	42.00	52.50	63.00	73.50	84.00
	1.46	2.13	36.20	38.30	40.50	42.60	53.30	63.90	74.60	85.00
4–10	1.47	2.16	36.70	38.80	41.00	43.20	54.00	64.80	75.60	86.00
	1.48	2.19	37.20	39.40	41.60	43.80	54.80	65.70	76.70	88.00
	1.49	2.22	37.70	40.00	42.20	44.40	55.50	66.60	77.70	89.00
4–11	1.50	2.25	38.30	40.50	42.80	45.00	56.30	67.50	78.80	90.00
	1.51	2.28	38.80	41.00	43.30	45.60	57.00	68.40	79.80	91.00
5–0	1.52	2.31	39.30	41.60	43.90	46.20	57.80	69.30	80.90	92.00
	1.53	2.34	39.80	42.10	44.50	46.80	58.50	70.20	81.90	94.00
	1.54	2.37	40.30	42.70	45.10	47.40	59.30	71.10	83.00	95.00
5–1	1.55	2.40	40.80	43.20	45.70	48.00	60.00	72.00	84.00	96.00
	1.56	2.43	41.30	43.70	46.20	48.60	60.80	72.90	85.10	97.00
	1.57	2.47	42.00	44.50	46.80	49.40	61.80	74.10	86.50	99.00
5–2	1.58	2.50	42.50	45.00	47.40	50.00	62.50	75.00	87.50	100.00
	1.59	2.53	43.00	43.00	48.00	50.60	63.25	75.90	88.60	101.00

5–3	1.60	2.56	43.50	46.10	48.60	51.20	64.00	76.80	89.60	102.00
	1.61	2.59	44.00	46.60	49.20	51.80	64.80	77.70	90.70	103.00
	1.62	2.62	44.50	47.20	49.90	52.40	65.50	78.60	91.70	105.00
5–4	1.63	2.66	45.20	47.90	50.50	53.20	66.50	79.80	93.10	106.00
	1.64	2.69	45.70	48.40	51.10	53.80	67.30	80.70	94.20	108.00
5–5	1.65	2.72	46.20	49.00	51.70	54.40	68.00	81.70	95.20	109.00
	1.66	2.76	46.90	49.70	52.40	55.20	69.00	82.80	96.60	110.00
	1.67	2.79	47.40	50.20	53.00	55.80	69.80	83.70	97.70	112.00
5–6	1.68	2.82	47.90	50.80	53.60	56.40	70.50	84.60	98.70	113.00
	1.69	2.86	48.60	51.50	54.30	57.20	71.50	85.80	100.10	114.00
5–7	1.70	2.89	49.10	52.00	54.90	57.80	72.30	86.70	101.20	116.00
	1.71	2.92	49.60	52.60	55.60	58.40	73.00	87.60	102.20	117.00
	1.72	2.96	50.30	53.30	56.20	59.20	74.00	88.80	103.60	118.00
5–8	1.73	2.99	50.80	53.30	56.80	59.80	74.80	89.70	104.70	120.00
	1.74	3.03	51.50	54.50	57.50	60.60	75.80	91.00	106.10	121.00
5–9	1.75	3.06	52.00	55.10	58.20	61.20	76.50	91.80	107.10	122.00
	1.76	3.10	52.70	55.80	58.90	62.00	77.50	93.00	108.50	124.00
	1.77	3.13	53.20	56.30	59.50	62.60	78.30	94.00	109.60	125.00
5–10	1.78	3.17	53.90	57.10	60.20	63.40	79.30	95.10	111.00	127.00
	1.79	3.20	54.50	57.60	60.80	64.00	80.00	96.00	112.00	128.00

(continued)

BMI CHARTS *(continued)*

Height (ft–in)	Height (m)	Height² (m²)	BMI 17 (kg)	BMI 18 (kg)	BMI 19 (kg)	BMI 20 (kg)	BMI 25 (kg)	BMI 30 (kg)	BMI 35 (kg)	BMI 40 (kg)
5–11	1.80	3.24	55.10	58.30	61.60	64.80	81.00	97.20	113.40	130.00
	1.81	3.28	55.76	59.04	62.32	65.60	82.00	98.00	115.00	131.00
	1.82	3.31	56.27	59.58	62.89	66.20	82.75	99.00	116.00	132.00
6–0	1.83	3.35	56.95	60.30	63.65	67.00	83.75	100.50	117.00	134.00
	1.84	3.38	57.46	60.84	64.22	67.60	84.50	101.00	118.00	135.00
	1.85	3.42	58.14	61.56	64.98	68.40	85.50	103.00	120.00	137.00
6–1	1.86	3.46	58.82	62.28	65.74	69.20	86.50	104.00	121.00	138.00
	1.87	3.50	59.50	63.00	66.50	70.00	87.50	105.00	123.00	140.00
6–2	1.88	3.53	60.01	63.54	67.07	70.60	88.25	106.00	124.00	141.00
	1.89	3.57	60.69	64.26	67.83	71.40	89.25	107.00	125.00	142.00
	1.90	3.61	61.37	64.78	68.59	72.20	90.25	108.00	126.00	144.00
6–3	1.91	3.65	62.05	65.71	69.35	73.00	91.25	110.00	128.00	146.00

BMI = weight (kg) ÷ height (m)²

Appendix B

Pounds to kilograms chart

POUNDS TO KILOGRAMS

Pounds	kg	Pounds	kg	Pounds	kg	Pounds	kg
1 lb	0.45 kg	50 lb	22.7 kg	99 lb	44.9 kg	148 lb	67.0 kg
2 lb	0.91 kg	51 lb	23.1 kg	100 lb	45.3 kg	149 lb	67.4 kg
3 lb	1.36 kg	52 lb	23.6 kg	101 lb	45.7 kg	150 lb	67.9 kg
4 lb	1.81 kg	53 lb	24.0 kg	102 lb	46.2 kg	151 lb	68.4 kg
5 lb	2.27 kg	54 lb	24.5 kg	103 lb	46.7 kg	152 lb	68.8 kg
6 lb	2.72 kg	55 lb	24.9 kg	104 lb	47.1 kg	153 lb	69.2 kg
7 lb	3.18 kg	56 lb (4 st)	25.4 kg	105 lb	47.6 kg	154 lb (11 st)	69.7 kg
8 lb	3.63 kg	57 lb	25.9 kg	106 lb	48.0 kg	155 lb	70.2 kg
9 lb	4.08 kg	58 lb	26.3 kg	107 lb	48.5 kg	156 lb	70.6 kg
10 lb	4.54 kg	59 lb	26.8 kg	108 lb	49.0 kg	157 lb	71.0 kg
11 lb	4.99 kg	60 lb	27.2 kg	109 lb	49.4 kg	158 lb	71.5 kg
12 lb	5.44 kg	61 lb	27.7 kg	110 lb	49.8 kg	159 lb	71.9 kg
13 lb	5.90 kg	62 lb	28.1 kg	111 lb	50.3 kg	160 lb	72.4 kg
14 lb (1 st)	6.35 kg	63 lb	28.6 kg	112 lb (8 st)	50.8 kg	161 lb	72.8 kg
15 lb	6.80 kg	64 lb	29.0 kg	113 lb	51.2 kg	162 lb	73.3 kg

lb	kg	lb	kg	lb	kg	lb	kg
16 lb	7.26 kg	65 lb	29.5 kg	114 lb	51.7 kg	163 lb	73.7 kg
17 lb	7.71 kg	66 lb	29.9 kg	115 lb	52.1 kg	164 lb	74.2 kg
18 lb	8.16 kg	67 lb	30.4 kg	116 lb	52.6 kg	165 lb	74.6 kg
19 lb	8.62 kg	68 lb	30.8 kg	117 lb	53.0 kg	166 lb	75.1 kg
20 lb	9.07 kg	69 lb	31.3 kg	118 lb	53.5 kg	167 lb	75.5 kg
21 lb	9.52 kg	70 lb (5 st)	31.7 kg	119 lb	53.9 kg	168 lb (12 st)	76.0 kg
22 lb	9.98 kg	71 lb	32.1 kg	120 lb	54.4 kg	169 lb	76.4 kg
23 lb	10.43 kg	72 lb	32.6 kg	121 lb	54.9 kg	170 lb	76.9 kg
24 lb	10.89 kg	73 lb	33.0 kg	122 lb	55.3 kg	171 lb	77.4 kg
25 lb	11.34 kg	74 lb	33.5 kg	123 lb	55.7 kg	172 lb	77.8 kg
26 lb	11.79 kg	75 lb	34.0 kg	124 lb	56.2 kg	173 lb	78.3 kg
27 lb	12.25 kg	76 lb	34.4 kg	125 lb	56.5 kg	174 lb	78.7 kg
28 lb (2 st)	12.70 kg	77 lb	34.8 kg	126 lb (9 st)	57.1 kg	175 lb	79.2 kg
29 lb	13.2 kg	78 lb	35.3 kg	127 lb	57.5 kg	176 lb	79.6 kg
30 lb	13.6 kg	79 lb	35.8 kg	128 lb	58.0 kg	177 lb	80.0 kg
31 lb	14.1 kg	80 lb	36.3 kg	129 lb	58.4 kg	178 lb	80.5 kg

(continued)

POUNDS TO KILOGRAMS (continued)

Pounds	kg	Pounds	kg	Pounds	kg	Pounds	kg
32 lb	14.5 kg	81 lb	36.7 kg	130 lb	58.9 kg	179 lb	80.9 kg
33 lb	15.0 kg	82 lb	37.3 kg	131 lb	59.3 kg	180 lb	81.4 kg
34 lb	15.4 kg	83 lb	37.6 kg	132 lb	59.8 kg	181 lb	81.8 kg
35 lb	15.9 kg	84 lb (6 st)	38.1 kg	133 lb	60.2 kg	182 lb (13 st)	82.3 kg
36 lb	16.3 kg	85 lb	38.5 kg	134 lb	60.7 kg	183 lb	82.7 kg
37 lb	16.8 kg	86 lb	39.0 kg	135 lb	61.1 kg	184 lb	83.2 kg
38 lb	17.2 kg	87 lb	39.4 kg	136 lb	61.6 kg	185 lb	83.6 kg
39 lb	17.7 kg	88 lb	39.9 kg	137 lb	62.1 kg	186 lb	84.1 kg
40 lb	18.1 kg	89 lb	40.3 kg	138 lb	62.5 kg	187 lb	84.5 kg

lb	kg	lb	kg	lb	kg	lb	kg
41 lb	18.6 kg	90 lb	40.8 kg	139 lb	62.9 kg	188 lb	85.0 kg
42 lb (3 st)	19.0 kg	91 lb	41.2 kg	140 lb (10 st)	63.4 kg	189 lb	85.5 kg
43 lb	19.5 kg	92 lb	41.7 kg	141 lb	63.8 kg	190 lb	85.9 kg
44 lb	20.0 kg	93 lb	42.2 kg	142 lb	64.3 kg	191 lb	86.3 kg
45 lb	20.4 kg	94 lb	42.6 kg	143 lb	64.7 kg	192 lb	86.8 kg
46 lb	20.9 kg	95 lb	43.0 kg	144 lb	65.2 kg	193 lb	87.3 kg
47 lb	21.3 kg	96 lb	43.5 kg	145 lb	65.6 kg	194 lb	87.7 kg
48 lb	21.8 kg	97 lb	44.0 kg	146 lb	66.1 kg	195 lb	88.2 kg
49 lb	22.2 kg	98 lb (7 st)	44.5 kg	147 lb	66.5 kg	196 lb (14 st)	88.6 kg

Appendix C

Quality of life: eating disorders (QOL ED) questionnaire

1. What is your:

   Current height (metres) _____

   Current weight (kg) _____

   Current BMI: (calculated) _____

2. On how many days did you ATTEMPT to LIMIT what you ate for any reason?

   In the PAST 28 days:

   0 days   1–7 days   8–14 days   15–21 days   22–28 days

3. On how many days did being PREOCCUPIED with thoughts of FOOD or EATING affect your concentration on other things, e.g. reading?

   In the PAST 28 days:

   0 days   1–7 days   8–14 days   15–21 days   22–28 days

4. On how many days did you want to feel EMPTY inside (for any reason)?

   In the PAST 28 days:

   0 days   1–7 days   8–14 days   15–21 days   22–28 days

5. Did you feel CONFUSED about what emotions you were feeling?

   In the PAST 28 days:

   not at all   a little   somewhat   moderately   a lot

6. Did you feel UNEASY attending social situations?

In the PAST 28 days:

not at all   a little   somewhat   moderately   a lot

7. Did you feel AFRAID of losing control over your body?

In the PAST 28 days:

not at all   a little   somewhat   moderately   a lot

8. Did you feel UNHAPPY and unable to cope as well as usual?

In the PAST 28 days:

not at all   a little   somewhat   moderately   a lot

9. Did you feel you had to do things PERFECTLY or you would have failed?

In the PAST 28 days:

not at all   a little   somewhat   moderately   a lot

10. On how many days did you feel AFRAID of losing control over your feelings?

In the PAST 28 days:

0 days   1–7 days   8–14 days   15–21 days   22–28 days

11. On how many days did you feel AFRAID of losing control over your eating?

In the PAST 28 days:

0 days   1–7 days   8–14 days   15–21 days   22–28 days

12. On how many days did you overeat?

In the PAST 28 days:

0 days   1–7 days   8–14 days   15–21 days   22–28 days

13. On how many days did you vomit?

    In the PAST 28 days:

    0 days   1–7 days   8–14 days   15–21 days   22–28 days

14. On how many days did you misuse laxatives?

    In the PAST 28 days:

    0 days   1–7 days   8–14 days   15–21 days   22–28 days

15. On how many days did being PREOCCUPIED with thoughts of BODY WEIGHT or SHAPE affect your concentration on other things, e.g. reading?

    In the PAST 28 days:

    0 days   1–7 days   8–14 days   15–21 days   22–28 days

A. What weight would you like to be? _____ kg (calculate desired BMI)

16. How important is exercise as a means of burning up energy or controlling your SHAPE or WEIGHT?

    In the PAST 28 days:

    not at all   a little   somewhat   moderately   a lot

17. How important is exercise to feel better MENTALLY, to prevent changes in mood, to assist with stress, or promote a sense of achievement?

    In the PAST 28 days:

    not at all   a little   somewhat   moderately   a lot

18. Has your CURRENT medical health been NEGATIVELY AFFECTED by your eating, exercise or body weight? (Include acute (short-term) problems that are expected to recover with treatment, change in body weight, or behaviour, e.g. low blood pressure, cardiac irregularities, electrolyte disturbances, fainting, low blood iron, dehydration.)

    In the PAST 28 days:

    not at all   a little   somewhat   moderately   a lot

B. Has your CONTINUING medical health been NEGATIVELY AFFECTED by your eating, exercise or body weight? (Include chronic (long-term) conditions that require ongoing management, medication, or have resulted in permanent changes, e.g. diabetes, impaired vision, renal damage, osteoporosis, infertility, dental problems)

In the PAST 28 days:

not at all   a little   somewhat   moderately   a lot

19. Has your STUDY, CAREER or WORK been negatively affected by your eating, exercise, or body weight?

In the PAST 28 days:

not at all   a little   somewhat   moderately   a lot

20. Have your SOCIAL LIFE or SOCIAL ACTIVITIES been negatively affected by your eating, exercise, or body weight?

In the PAST 28 days:

not at all   a little   somewhat   moderately   a lot

21. Have your RELATIONSHIPS with family and friends been negatively affected by your eating, exercise or body weight?

In the PAST 28 days:

not at all   a little   somewhat   moderately   a lot

22. Did you try to follow SPECIFIC rules regarding your exercise or activity, e.g. I must do a certain number of laps, minutes, or circuits, and NOT general guidelines?

In the PAST 28 days:

0 days   1–7 days   8–14 days   15–21 days   22–28 days

23. Would you feel UNHAPPY and DISTRESSED if you were unable to exercise when you wanted?

In the PAST 28 days:

0 days   1–7 days   8–14 days   15–21 days   22–28 days

24. Did you feel like a BAD PERSON if you did not exercise a certain amount?

In the PAST 28 days:

0 days   1–7 days   8–14 days   15–21 days   22–28 days

25. Did you feel you HAD TO exercise?

In the PAST 28 days:

0 days   1–7 days   8–14 days   15–21 days   22–28 days

26. Did being PREOCCUPIED with thoughts of EXERCISE affect your concentration on other things?

In the PAST 28 days:

0 days   1–7 days   8–14 days   15–21 days   22–28 days

27. Did you feel AFRAID of losing CONTROL over your exercise?

In the PAST 28 days:

0 days   1–7 days   8–14 days   15–21 days   22–28 days

28. Did you feel uneasy if you did not have access to food or know where food is available?

In the PAST 28 days:

not at all   a little   somewhat   moderately   a lot

29. Did you eat food to feel better MENTALLY, e.g. to promote a feeling of well-being or to decrease feelings of tension or stress?

In the PAST 28 days:

not at all   a little   somewhat   moderately   a lot

30. Did you feel you wanted to EAT MORE food than you did?

In the PAST 28 days:

0 days   1–7 days   8–14 days   15–21 days   22–28 days

31. On how many days did you binge eat?

    In the PAST 28 days:

    0 days   1–7 days   8–14 days   15–21 days   22–28 days

32. Did you want to feel FULL inside (for any reason)?

    In the PAST 28 days:

    0 days   1–7 days   8–14 days   15–21 days   22–28 days

Scoring QOL ED

1. Body weight score:

   BMI:

> 40	4
35–39.9	3
30–34.9	2
25–29.9	1
19–24.9	0
18–18.9	1
17–17.9	2
15–16.9	3
<15	4

2. Eating behaviour score:

   Questions: total 2+12+13+14+(highest score of question 16 or 17) converted to 0–4 scale (0=0, 1–5=1, 6–10=2, 11–15=3, 16–20=4)

3. Eating disorder scale:

   Questions: total 3+4+7+11+15 converted to 0–4 scale (0=0, 1–5=1, 6–10=2, 11–15=3, 16–20=4)

4. Psychological score:

   Questions: total 5+6+8+9+10 converted to 0–4 scale (0=0, 1–5=1, 6–10=2, 11–15=3, 16–20=4)

5. Daily living score:

   Questions: 19+20+21 converted to 0–4 scale (0=0, 1–3=1, 4–6=2, 7–9=3, 10–12=4)

6. Acute medical score:

   Question: 18

7. Global score:

   Total of all six domain scores above (0–4), total score 0–24

8. Exercise:

   Questions: total 22+23+24+25+26+27 converted to 0–4 scale (0=0, 1–5=1, 6–10=2, 11–15=3, 16–20=4)

9. Overeating:

   Questions: total 28+29+30+31+32+33 converted to 0–4 scale (0=0, 1–5=1, 6–10=2, 11–15=3, 16–20=4)

10. Chronic medical score:

   Question: 18 B

Quality of life QOL ED scores for eating disorder and non-eating-disordered women aged 15–35 years (average scores and scores for 50% of women)

QOL scores[a]	Patients with eating disorders		Control women	
	Average	95%	Average	95%
Global	14.9	14.0–15.8	5.0	4.6–5.4
Body weight	2.1	1.7–2.5	0.4	0.3–0.5
Eating behaviour	1.7	1.5–1.8	1.2	1.1–1.3
Eating disorder	2.2	2.0–2.3	1.1	1.0–1.2
Overeating feelings	1.9	1.8–2.1	1.2	1.1–1.3
Exercise feelings	2.3	2.1–2.5	1.5	1.4–1.6
Psychological feelings	3.2	3.0–3.5	1.2	1.1–1.3
Daily living	3.0	2.7–3.2	0.75	0.6–0.90
Acute medical	2.3	1.9–2.6	0.33	0.2–0.4

[a] Lower scores indicate a better quality of life.
(*Australian and New Zealand Journal of Psychiatry* 2006; **40**: 150–5.)

Glossary

Adipose tissue The tissues of the body that contain numbers of fat cells. Adipose tissue is 80% fat, 2% protein, and 18% water. Because of the large proportion of fat, adipose tissue is often called fatty tissue.

Alkalosis An increase in the alkalinity of the blood, which normally is slightly acidic. It is usually due to an increase in the level of bicarbonate in the blood.

Amenorrhoea The cessation or absence of menstruation for more than 3 months.

Amniotic fluid The fluid that surrounds the fetus during pregnancy, providing protection, room to move and develop, and a constant temperature; it is essential for lung development.

Anorexia nervosa See page 24 for diagnostic criteria.

Asperger's disorder An autism spectrum disorder associated with difficulties in social, emotional and communication skills and good rote memory.

Assisted conception An intervention that manipulates the egg and/or the sperm to produce a pregnancy. It may include the use of drugs, hormones, *in vitro* fertilization (IVF) or any number of newer technologies.

Average body weight (ABW) The average body weight for age, height, and weight.

Bariatrics A branch of medicine involved with treating obesity.

Behaviour therapy A psychological therapy based on experimental psychology, intended to change symptoms and behaviour by various techniques, for example, anxiety management training, assertiveness training, aversion therapy, biofeedback, and desensitization.

Body mass index (BMI) A measure devised over 100 years ago to determine whether a person is of normal weight, underweight, or obese (pages 22 and 36).

Bulimia nervosa See page 29 for definition.

Calories A lay term for kilocalories (see entry for kilocalories).

237

Carbohydrates The class of nutrients made up of starches and sugars. Carbohydrates provide the main source of energy needed for the human body to function. Starches are the most common form of dietary carbohydrate and are found in cereal grains, roots, and tubers. In the human gut, starches are broken down to sugars and finally to glucose, which is absorbed into the blood.

Carotenaemia Condition in which the skin turns a yellow colour, usually from an increased dietary intake of carotenoids (e.g. carrots).

Chyme Liquid substance formed in the stomach when partially digested food is mixed with hydrochloric acid and digestive enzymes.

Cognitive behavioural therapy Psychological therapy intended to change maladaptive ways of thinking and thereby bring about improvement in psychological disorders.

Cortisol A steroid hormone released by the body in response to stress.

Diuretics Drugs that act on the kidney to increase the flow of urine.

Dizygotic Twins formed as a result of two eggs being fertilized by different sperm and embedded in the uterine wall at the same time.

Dyspepsia Persistent pain in the upper abdomen, which can also manifest as abdominal fullness or feeling full faster than expected when eating.

Dysphoric unpleasant mood, e.g. depressed or anxious.

Eclampsia Severe pregnancy-induced hypertension, characterized by seizures, coma, hypertension, proteinuria (protein in the urine), and oedema. Causes complications during delivery and can result in the death of the fetus and mother.

Electrolyte A substance that, when dissolved in water, separates into electrically charged particles (ions) capable of conducting an electrical current, e.g. sodium, potassium, chloride.

Endocannabinoids Substances produced by the body that activate cannabinoid receptors in the brain.

Follicle-stimulating hormone (FSH) A hormone secreted by the pituitary gland that stimulates growth of the egg follicles in the ovary and development of sperm in the testis.

Gestational diabetes mellitus An inability of the mother to metabolize carbohydrates during pregnancy, usually due to a deficiency in insulin. In most women, the condition disappears after pregnancy.

Ghrenlin A hormone that stimulates appetite via activation of neuropeptide Y.

Glucose A simple sugar found in food; the major source of energy for humans.

Glycogen The form in which sugars and starches are stored in animals. Sucrose and starches from plants are converted into glucose before being absorbed into the human body from the gut, and the glucose is converted into glycogen for storage in the liver and in muscle.

Heart rate Normal heart rate is within the range of 60–80 beats per minute.

Hernia Protrusion of a tissue structure through the membrane or muscular tissue that normally contains it.

Hyperemesis gravidarum A rare condition of pregnancy characterized by protracted vomiting, weight loss, dehydration, and an imbalance of electrolytes requiring treatment in hospital.

Hyperlipidaemia When the level of lipids (e.g. cholesterol and triglycerides) in the blood is too high.

Hypertension High blood pressure.

Hypothalamus The part of the brain just above the brain stem that controls the activity of the pituitary gland.

Insulin A hormone secreted by the pancreas to promote entry of glucose into the liver and muscles where it is stored as glycogen.

Insulin-like growth factor A hormone thought to be regulated by nutrition that is required for growth and development of the fetus.

Kilocalorie A kilocalorie (also called kcal, or calories) is a measure of the energy in foods. It is defined as the amount of heat required to raise the temperature of a litre of water from 15 to 16°C. Each food contains a different amount of energy, which is absorbed into the body after eating and expended to keep the body functioning. Recently, kcal have been replaced by a new energy measurement called a kilojoule (1 kcal = 4.19 kJ).

Kilojoule (kJ) Measure of energy, which has replaced the kilocalorie (1 kJ = 0.24 kcal).

Lanugo Soft, downy hair, similar to that found in small babies.

Laxatives Drugs that act on the bowel to increase the speed of the passage of food and of stools through the gut. They cause soft and frequent motions.

Leptin A hormone secreted from adipose tissue with a key role in regulating energy intake by signalling satiety. Blood levels of leptin are a measure of body fatness.

Libido A person's sexual desire, arousal, and awareness.

Luteinizing hormone (LH) A hormone secreted by and released from the pituitary gland that leads to the release of a mature egg (or ovum) from an ovarian follicle and converts the follicle into a corpus luteum (or yellow body).

Menarche The onset of menstruation.

Millilitre (ml) Equivalent to 0.035 fluid ounces.

Monozygotic Twins formed from the same egg, which therefore have the same genetic profile.

Neuropeptide Y (NPY) A natural substance in the brain and autonomic nervous system that enhances appetite.

Neurotransmitter Brain chemicals that modify or relay signals between a neuron and another cell.

Noradrenaline A hormone released in response to stress that increases heart rate by triggering release of glucose from storage and increasing blood flow to muscles.

Obesity See page 36 for definition.

Oedema The accumulation of fluid in an organ or tissue space (swelling).

Opioids A chemical substance produced synthetically or endogenously, to provide pain relief.

Osteoarthritis Wear-and-tear damage of the bone and cartilage in a joint producing inflammation, pain, and limitation of movement.

Osteopenia A decrease in bone mineral density; a precursor to osteoporosis.

Osteoporosis Low bone mineral density (2.5 standard deviations below peak bone mass) in which the microarchitecture of the bone is disrupted and the bone is weakened.

Ovaries The pair of female reproductive organs that produce and release an egg from the follicle (on the ovary surface). This process occurs each month, under the guidance of follicle-stimulating hormone and luteinizing hormone.

Peristalsis The wave-like, progressive, sequential movement of the wall of the intestines, which churns up food and moves it on towards the anus.

Picking behaviour Moving from food in the cupboard, to the pantry, to the fridge, to pick and eat small quantities of various foods.

Pituitary gland The gland located at the base of the brain that affects the function of other glands by releasing special hormones.

Placebo A harmless substance administered to test the effectiveness of an active substance in a scientific study.

Placenta Highly vascularized organ of pregnancy that allows exchange of nutrients, gases, and waste products between the fetus and the mother.

Polycystic ovarian syndrome Hormonal disorder occurring in women; primarily features irregular or lack of menstrual bleeding, problems with weight control, and effects of masculinizing hormones (e.g. hair growth in male patterns).

Postpartum After child birth.

Quetelet Index See body mass index.

Resistance behaviour Behaviour used as a method of stopping abnormal eating patterns.

Resting metabolic rate The resting metabolic rate can be calculated from the formula:

$$RMR = 99.8 \ (\text{body weight in kg} \times 1.155) + (\text{total body potassium} \times 0.0223) - (\text{age} \times 0.456)$$

The result is expressed as the oxygen uptake in ml/minute. If this figure is multiplied by 7, a rough approximation of the energy expenditure (in kcal) is obtained.

Satiety (satiation) The feeling of 'fullness' after eating food.

Serotonin A neurotransmitter in the brain, believed to have a number of roles in mood, sexuality, anger, body temperature, vomiting, and sleep.

Social anxiety (social phobia) Anxiousness in social situations, which causes distress and hinders the person's everyday life; an intense fear of being judged by others and of embarrassment or humiliation by the person's own actions.

Steatohepatitis Inflammation with concurrent fat deposition in the liver.

Testicles The pair of male reproductive organs that produce sperm and the hormone testosterone.

Tryptophan An essential amino acid (i.e. cannot be synthesized by the body, so it must be derived from the diet), used to make proteins in the body; it is a precursor for other substances (e.g. serotonin).

Withdrawal bleed A 'fake period', which happens to women who are on the contraceptive pill. The monthly bleeding is due to cessation of the hormones provided by the pill, and no ovulation occurs.

Index